Carolyn's journey through breast cancer as chronicled by her husband

"I'm not a fighter, I'm just tough" – Carolyn

Christopher Bidwell

Printed in the United States of America
Illustrations by Christopher Bidwell

First Printing, 2015

Library of Congress Cataloging-in-Publication data available.

ISBN 978-0-692-52183-0

IngramSpark Publishing
1 Ingram Blvd
La Vergne, Tennessee
(877) 997-7275
http://www.ingramspark.com/

This book is dedicated to the staff at Anschutz Hospital, particularly her doctors and the nurses in the Breast Cancer Center.

Doctor Kabos was Carolyn's Oncologist and was extremely supportive and open. He was very good about laying out our options with the pros and cons and giving us his advice on which avenue of treatment to pursue but leaving the actual choice up to us.

I would also like to acknowledge the wonderful nurses and staff in the Infusion Center, in particular the RNs Stacy and Nichole, the staff Christina and Carol and our favorite CNA Sasha.

Carolyn had a close relationship with them all.

This book is also dedicated to Carolyn's daughter Hailey. She and Carolyn talked, texted and supported each other on a daily basis during the entire period that Carolyn had cancer. In fact during this period, their relationship grew to include best friends as part of the mother-daughter connection.

Contents

Preface

This project started several months before Carolyn, my wife passed away from Metastatic breast cancer as a way to give an insight into what we went through during our on again, off again battle with cancer. The project started as drawings in a notebook and eventually I started creating them digitally on my iPad so that I could post them on Facebook for our friends and family to see. The project then grew to provide some insight for women who are currently fighting cancer, those that have been recently diagnosed with cancer and their friends and family as well. Since most of these people are not my friends on Facebook, the project took a turn into becoming a book.

I have tried to be honest, truthful and open with all the insights as Carolyn and I experienced them. They are mostly presented in the order that they were created. The drawings get more and more refined as they go along since I learned quite a bit about creating them as I went along.

When Carolyn was initially diagnosed with inflammatory breast cancer because the initial source of the cancer was so close to the skin, but they later changed that diagnosis since she never had any skin lesions. At that time we were completely ignorant of what would be involved in her treatment. We were using a new set of doctors that we did not know, we did not know what was involved with the chemo therapy, the medications, the scans and equipment, the changes to our lives, how our emotions would do in dealing with the disease, what surgeries or radiation would be involved, would she lose her hair, and so many other unknowns. I had two main reasons for continuing these insights after her death. The first is to shed light and provide an insight into some of these unknowns. Knowledge is power and a little insight into what is coming up can help you to make better decisions and to make the whole process a little less scary. The second is a celebration of Carolyn's incredible life, what she went through during her years fighting cancer and it is a way for me to deal with the grief of her death.

From several of the insights, you might think that we were against chemotherapy, but exactly the opposite is the case. Carolyn's chemotherapy gave her another two or three years of life and those were the best years of my life and some of the best of

Carolyn's life as well. We will be forever indebted to our incredible Oncologist and the extremely talented and compassionate nurses in the Cancer Center and the Infusion Center.

These insights are based on the six years and 5 months that Carolyn (Carrie) Bidwell and I were fighting her breast cancer together. These are all based on things that we went through or learned from our experiences and from talking to our doctors and nurses.

Her treatment in a nutshell

1. First Chemo phase (16 months) - Carolyn was initially diagnosed with breast cancer and we fought it with chemo and a unilateral mastectomy.
2. Cured (13 months) – Tests showed that Carolyn did not have any indications of breast cancer
3. Last Chemo phase (4 years) – Carolyn was diagnosed with metastatic breast cancer that is incurable and is treated as a chronic disease. Her cancer was diagnosed at this time as triple negative meaning the breast cancer cells tested negative for estrogen receptors (ER-), progesterone receptors (PR-), and HER2 (HER2-).
4. Carolyn passed away at the age of 58 on Wednesday, October 29th 2014.

Forward

This is a story of Carolyn and my cancer journey, so I should start at the beginning.

Carolyn always would get lumps in her breasts but they always turned out to be little cysts that could be drained so she would not be too alarmed if we felt a lump. We went into the doctor's office to have one of these drained and he could only get a little fluid out of it. We were not worried since he said that it was probably a fibroid, but he took a little biopsy just to be sure.

The following week, I was out of town on a business trip in San Francisco when I got a call on my first morning there just as I was about to go into a meeting. It was Carolyn and she told me that the results of the biopsy had come back and that she had breast cancer! I felt like I was punched in the stomach. I immediately left for the airport and flew home to be with her and figure out what we would do. We mostly hugged and talked about what would happen. We had no idea of what the treatment would be, what tests we would need, what new doctors we would be seeing. It was a whole new world that we new nothing about.

The story picks up in the page on "The First Day", but this story is not presented in chronological order, but in the order that they happened to pop into our heads as something important or interesting or even silly that we would not want to forget. I have to admit that I had a hard time finishing this book since it was my last really strong connection to Carolyn after she was gone.

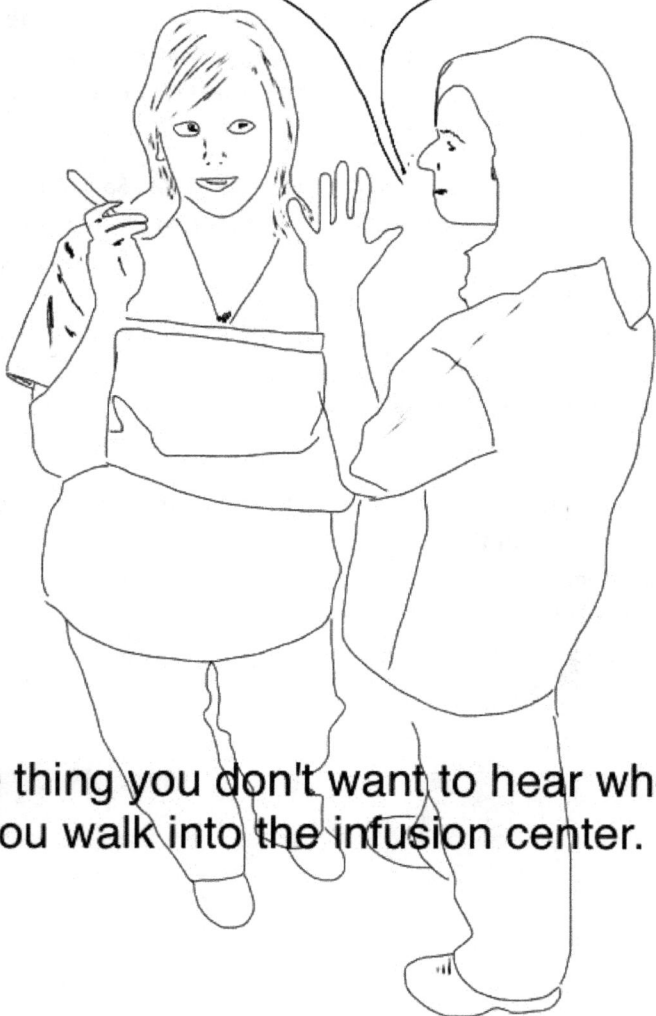

One thing you don't want to hear when you walk into the infusion center.

Carolyn currently has 18 prescriptions, not including the infusion drugs.

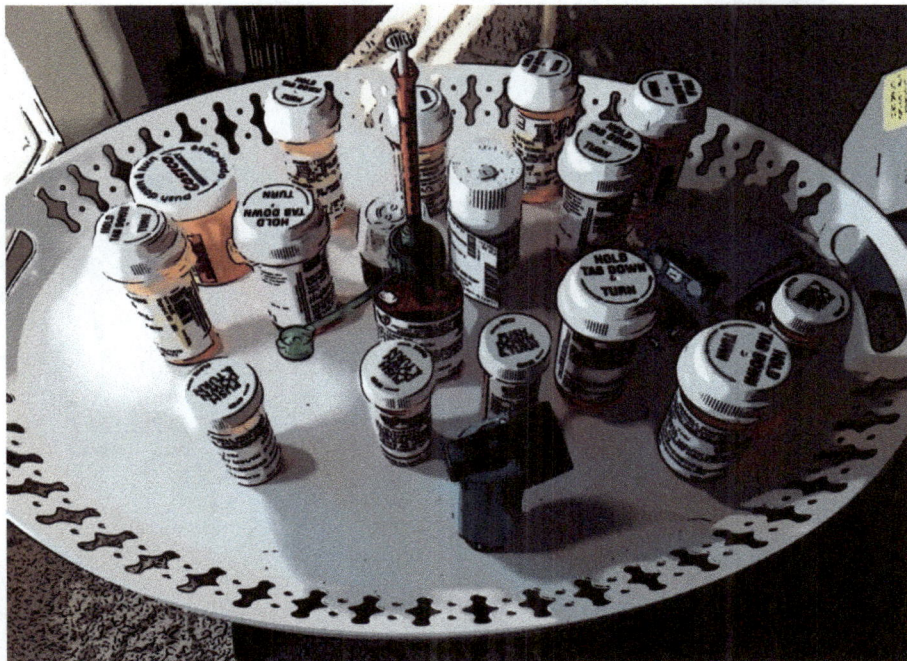

Her favorite drug however is her morning coffee.

Popping pills

When you are taking lots of pills every day, there is not time to take each one at a time. This calls for taking them a handful at a time. Be sure to have lots to drink, such as this refreshing iced tea.

Carolyn used the Lean Forward method. This is especially good for the larger capsule-style pills. Start by putting all the pills on your tongue. Take a medium sip and lean forward as you are swallowing the pills.
After the pills are down, continue with a couple of extra sips to ensure that none get stuck in your throat.

Many people have trouble swallowing pills. For them the only option is just to prolong the process by taking them one at a time.

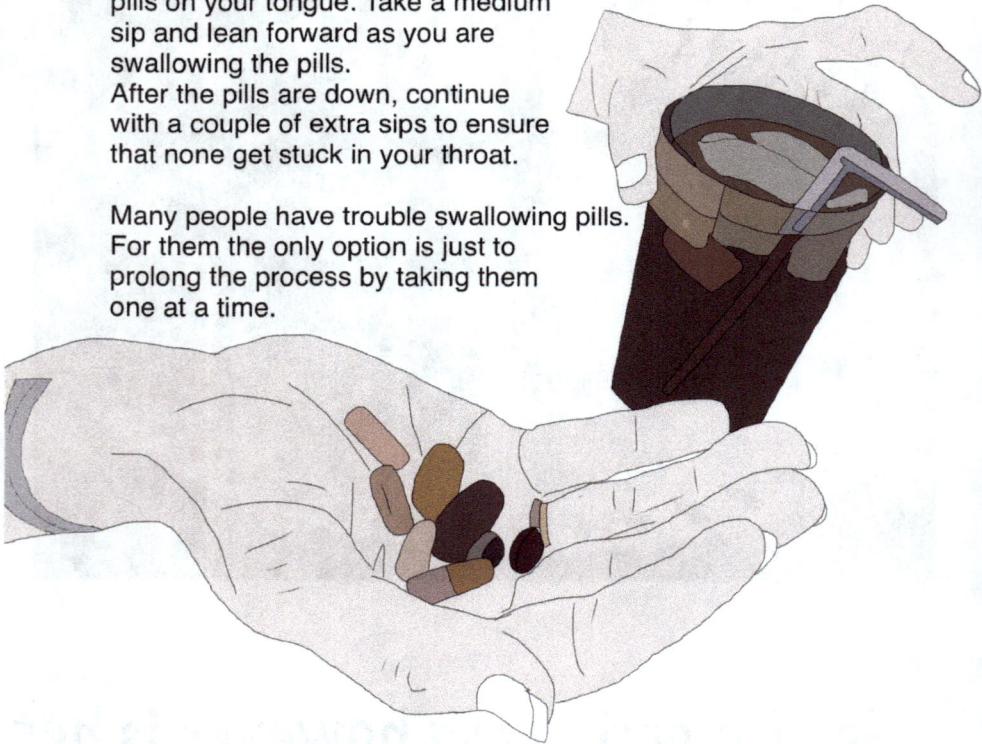

10 TOP

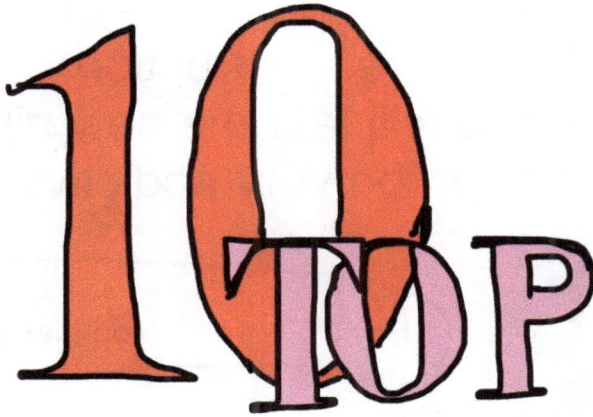

Carolyn's top ten things that are good about chemo/cancer

1) Don't have to shave your legs.
2) There really aren't any others baby.

After breast reconstruction,
the doctor will tattoo a new nipple.
Tattoos can be very addictive.

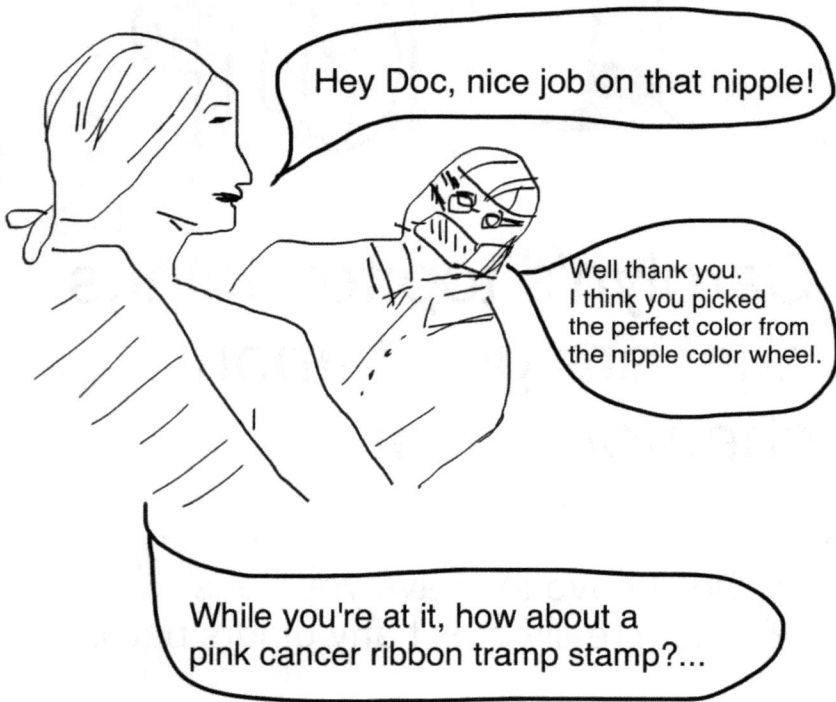

Hey Doc, nice job on that nipple!

Well thank you.
I think you picked
the perfect color from
the nipple color wheel.

While you're at it, how about a
pink cancer ribbon tramp stamp?...

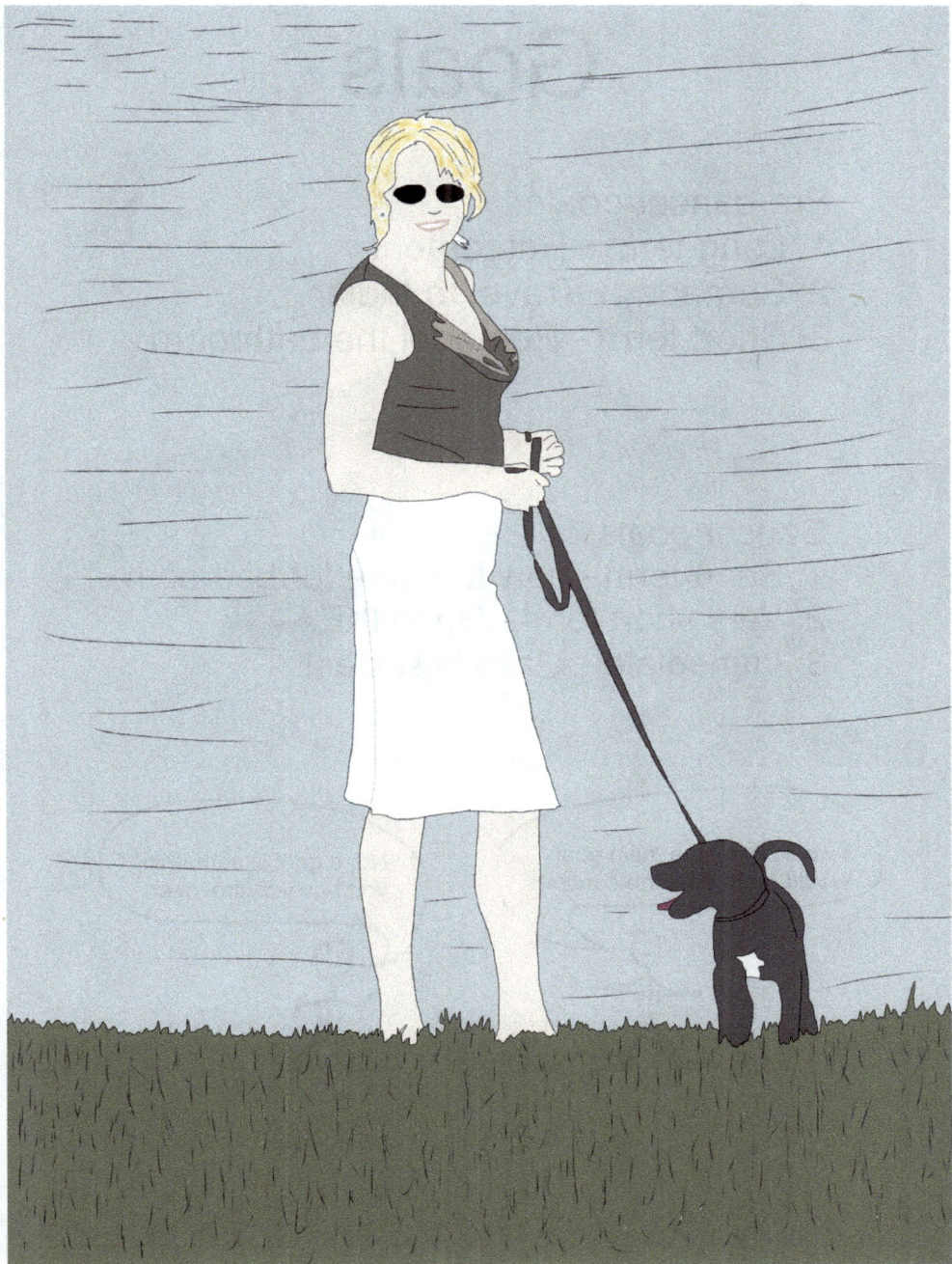

Goals

Pre-cancer goals
1. Long term - Retirement
2. Someday - Travel to India
3. Short term - Remodel the bathroom

Cancer goals
1. Short term - new furniture for bedroom
2. Very short term - Go to IKEA
3. Immediate - Make breakfast

I would think the main goal would be to beat the cancer!

No, a goal is something you have control over.

Perfect Health → → → No Health

Carolyn diagnosed with breast cancer, age 52

AC (Adriamycin & Cytoxan)

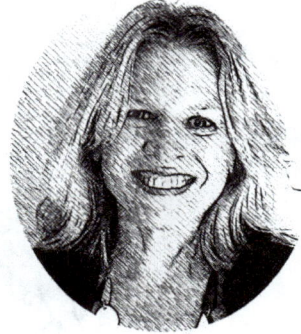

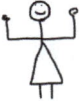

Taxol & Herceptin

Herceptin - only

Xeloda

Cured for a year, moved to foothills
Cancer came back, this time metastasized, age 54

Probable end of life without chemo, age 55

Navelbine

Gemzar

Your health takes a hit on each different chemo drug treatment.

Erubulin

Afinitor & Arimidex

Each time a new treatment is started, your body is a notch lower in health, energy and vitality.

Abraxane
Carolyn still fighting cancer, age 58

Targeted radiation treatment or "Spot Welding"

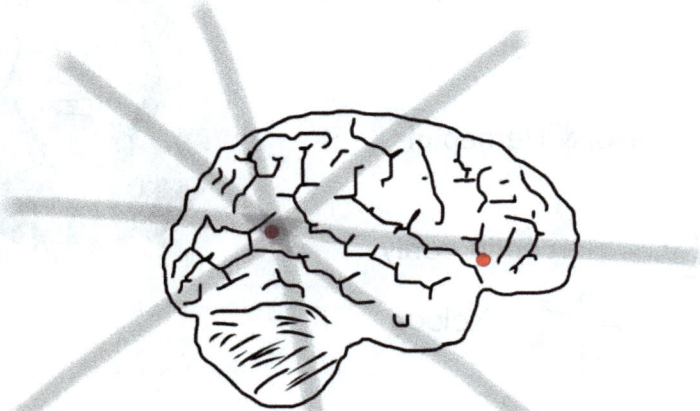

Up to 5 precisely targeted radiation beams coalesce on a single tumor, essentially vaporizing it while the surrounding tissue gets a relatively low dose.

Afterwards, you get a cool fiberglass cast of your head and shoulders that they used to bolt you to the table.

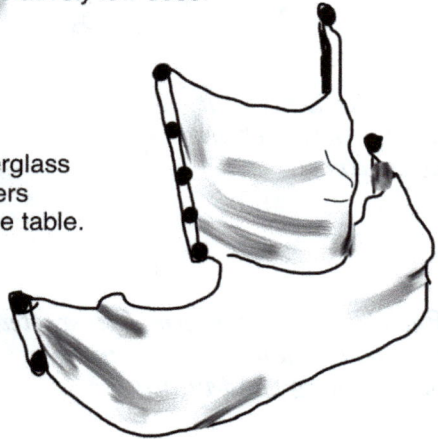

Chemo in a nutshell

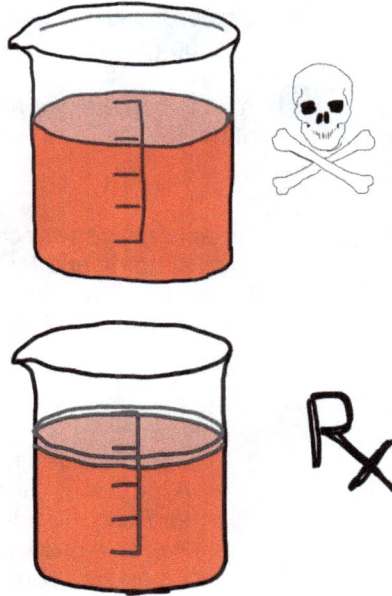

Figure out exactly how much will kill you.

Back off a little and infuse that amount.

In-Home Oxygen Systems

1.

8-16 hour supply
2-4 hour supply

Compressed air tanks for traveling and home Backup (power failures).

A 60 lb home oxygen concentrator is used at home

2.

8 hours with battery packs.

Portable oxygen concentrator.
Used at home and for traveling.
It uses 110 volt power, a car charger, and rechargeable battery packs.

3.

11 day supply

8 hour supply

Liquid oxygen tanks.
A large tank for home use and for filling the portable oxygen tanks.
Portable tanks for traveling.
An oxygen concentrator is mostly used at home

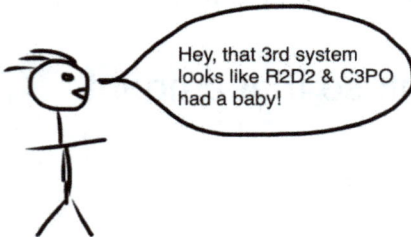

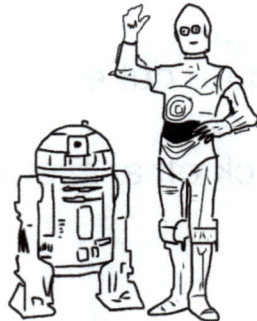

Hey, that 3rd system looks like R2D2 & C3PO had a baby!

Lung cancer from smoking vs lung cancer from metastatic breast cancer

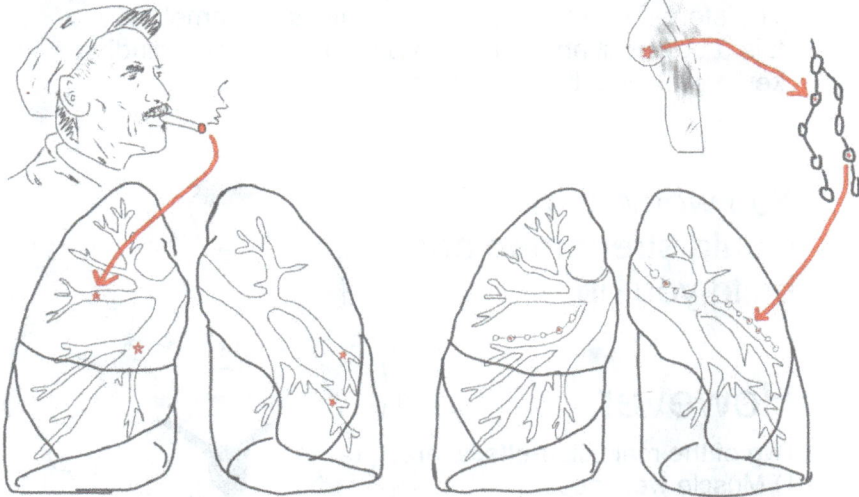

From smoking, the tumors start right in the lungs.

Breathing is difficult because The tumors are blocking the flow of air in the bronchial passages.

From metastatic breast cancer the tumor starts in the breast. It then spreads to the lymph system. Finally it creates tumors in the lymph nodes of the lungs.

Breathing is difficult because the lymphatic system prevents oxygen from getting into the blood stream.

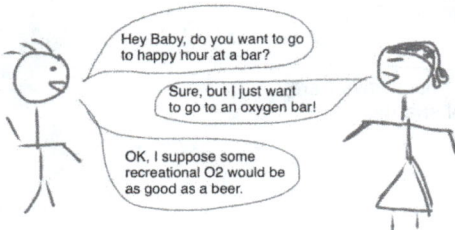

Steriods & Cancer

The steriod used for cancer patients is Dexamethasone. It is a powerful anti-inflammatory for the body including key organs like the brain and lungs.

You would think it would strengthen and build you up.

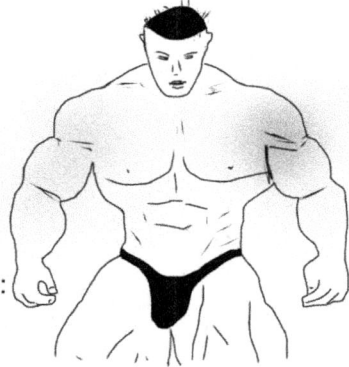

However

Two of the main side-effects are:
1) Muscle weakness
2) Loss of muscle mass
It is NOT an anabolic steroid.

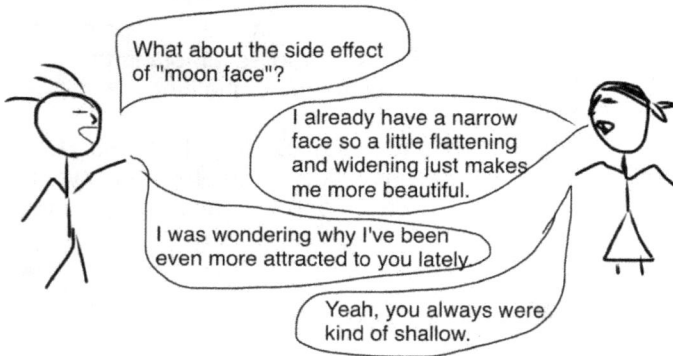

What about the side effect of "moon face"?

I already have a narrow face so a little flattening and widening just makes me more beautiful.

I was wondering why I've been even more attracted to you lately.

Yeah, you always were kind of shallow.

If you should not eat the foods that you like when on chemo, then what do you do when you are on Chemotherapy for life?

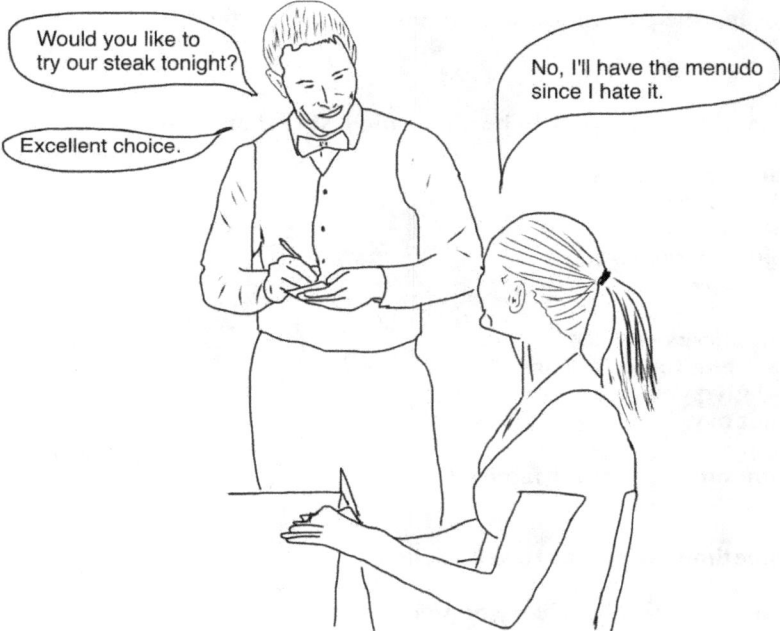

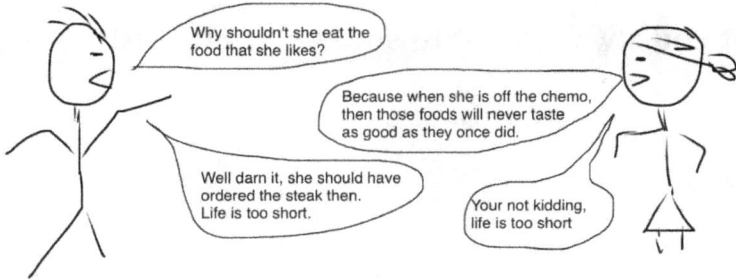

Cancer fatigue

Between the disease, the chemo, the anti-nausea drugs and the pain meds, sometimes you get fatigued.

Sometimes you want to be alone and just rest and relax.

Sometimes you want to just spend a quiet day with your husband enjoying each other's company.

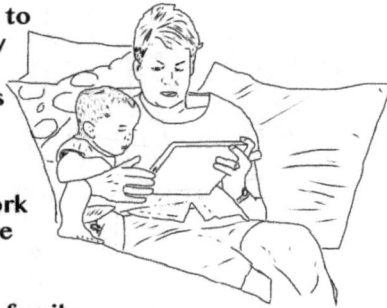

Sometimes you just want him to go to work and give you an entire quiet day.

Sometimes you want family to visit.

Sometimes you want to see friends.

Sometimes you feel like shopping.

But you always want to see the grandkids!

Chemo is the state of the art in cancer treatment, currently.

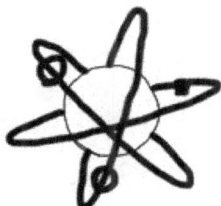

As Vince Masuka on Dexter said...

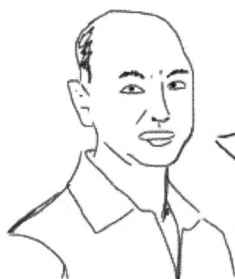

That's not opinion, that's science! Science is one cold hearted bitch

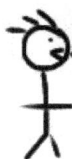

I wonder what chemo will Be like in 100 years?

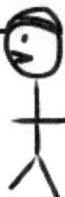

It will be like us looking back 200 years when the state of the art was draining the "bad" blood.

Infusion ports

3 little nubs help the nurse feel the port. The needle goes in the center of the nubs.

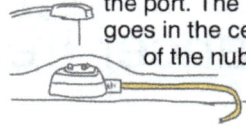

Chemo is very caustic and is hard on your veins.
In fact the veins in your arms where the infusion is delivered can become hardened and worn out.

The solution is an infusion port.
A port is surgically placed just under the skin.
The attached catheter goes up over the clavicle and into the jugular vein.

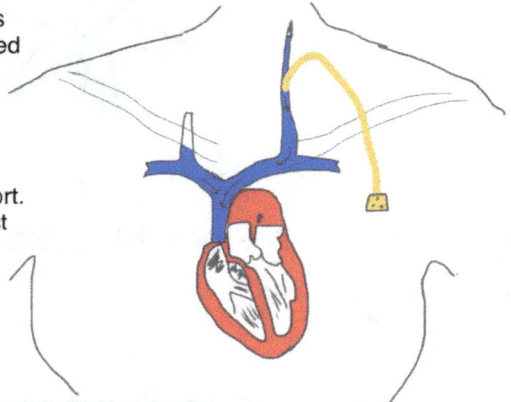

The idea is that the huge jugular will quickly disperse and dilute the chemo as it goes into the heart, preventing burning.
You also don't get tracks in your arm since the port is accessed in the same location each time.

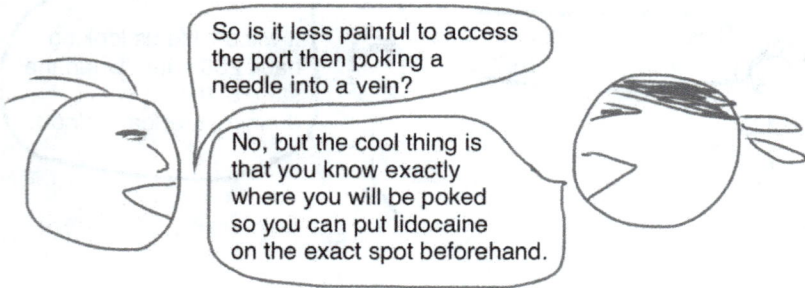

So is it less painful to access the port then poking a needle into a vein?

No, but the cool thing is that you know exactly where you will be poked so you can put lidocaine on the exact spot beforehand.

What do you have?

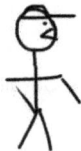

I have metastatic Breast cancer.

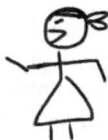

What is that?

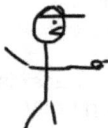

It means the cancer has spread to other parts of my body.

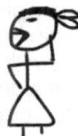

Is that bad?

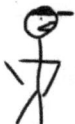

It's terminal, so we treat it as a chronic disease using chemo therapy for life.

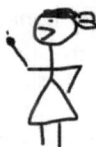

Oh sorry. So how soon can you quit the chemo treatments?

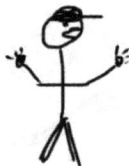

¿Arrrg!

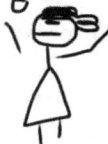

Tracking Cancer Growth

Discovering and diagnosing cancer is done with tools like mammograms, ultrasounds and biopsies. The tools listed below are what Oncologists use to track the progress of the disease and determine the best treatment.

MRI Magnetic Resonance Imaging. Much higher soft tissue detail than CT scan or X-Ray. No known hazards.

Using a strong magnetic field with radio waves, this causes tissues to emit their own radio waves. Different tissues have different chemical make-up and emit different intensities.

CT Scan Computer Tomography. Useful for detecting abnormal growth like tumors. Uses a series of X-Rays.

Takes continuous X-Ray pictures of the body a few mm apart like slices of bread. A contrast may be injected to help differentiate between organs and tumors.

PET Scan Positron Emmission Tomography. A radioactive tracer is injected. Useful for getting details of functioning body parts.

The tracer is basically radioactive sugar. Cancer cells absorb sugar more avidly, helping to locate tumors on the scan since they will "light up" on the images.

X-Ray Electromagnetic radiation particles. Can see some diseased tissue, but mostly for bones and lungs.

Different tissues absorb different amounts of radiation. Bones appear white while fat and soft tissues are gray.

Blood test Look for tumor markers which are chemicals made by tumor cells.

Although not foolproof tumor markers can be used to track the response to treatment.

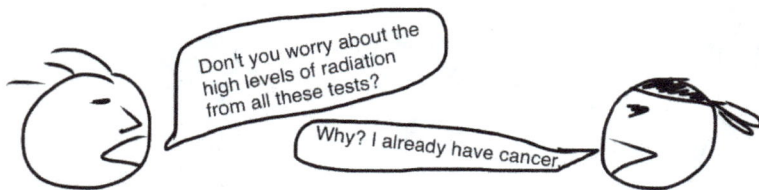

Don't you worry about the high levels of radiation from all these tests?

Why? I already have cancer.

BRCA Gene

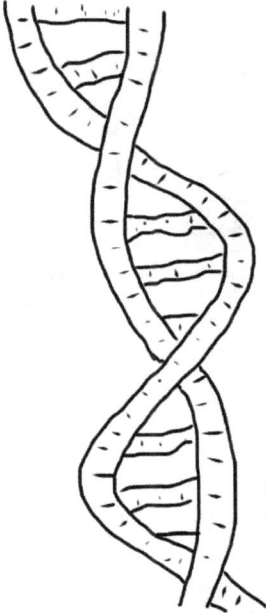

Normal BRCA genes repair damaged genes, repair damaged DNA or destroy genes that are beyond repair.

The problem is abnormal mutations of the BRCA gene, not the gene itself.

The BRCA test is a DNA test that looks for these mutations.

Women with this mutation have a 3 to 7 times greater risk of getting breast cancer than those without.

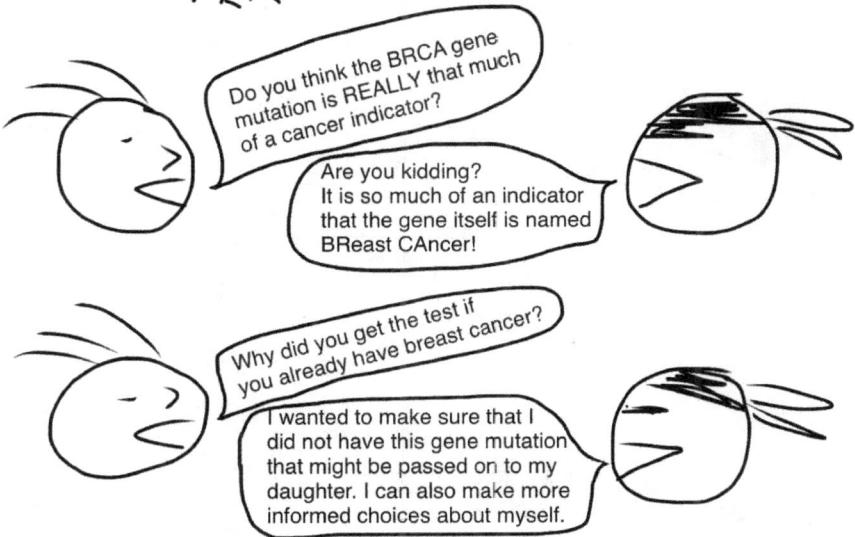

Do you think the BRCA gene mutation is REALLY that much of a cancer indicator?

Are you kidding? It is so much of an indicator that the gene itself is named BReast CAncer!

Why did you get the test if you already have breast cancer?

I wanted to make sure that I did not have this gene mutation that might be passed on to my daughter. I can also make more informed choices about myself.

White Blood Cell Count

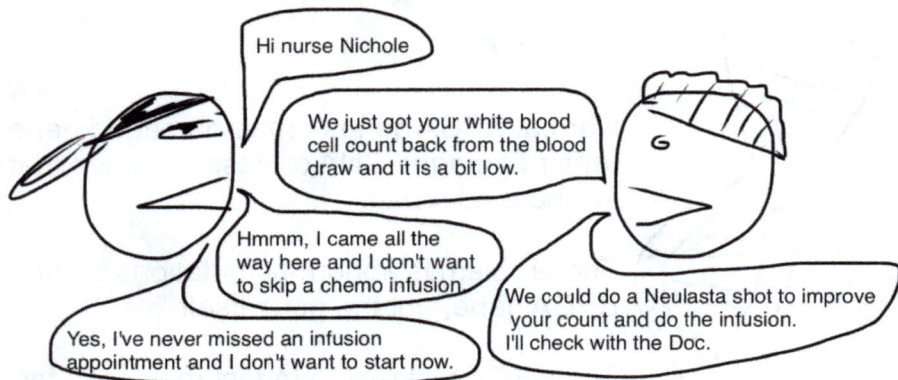

Hi nurse Nichole

We just got your white blood cell count back from the blood draw and it is a bit low.

Hmmm, I came all the way here and I don't want to skip a chemo infusion.

Yes, I've never missed an infusion appointment and I don't want to start now.

We could do a Neulasta shot to improve your count and do the infusion. I'll check with the Doc.

A side-effect of chemo is a decrease in white blood cells. These cells help fight infection and a low count puts you at risk for developing infections.

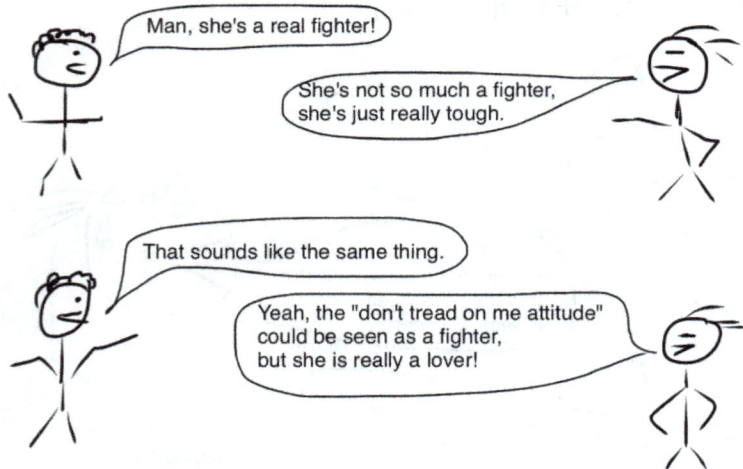

Man, she's a real fighter!

She's not so much a fighter, she's just really tough.

That sounds like the same thing.

Yeah, the "don't tread on me attitude" could be seen as a fighter, but she is really a lover!

The PET Scan

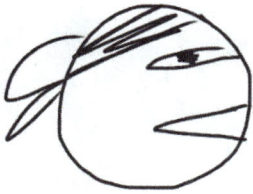

The PET scan is the King of the scans. This scan of a tumor near my right bronchial passage shows why.

Same tumor 14 weeks later

Original tumor

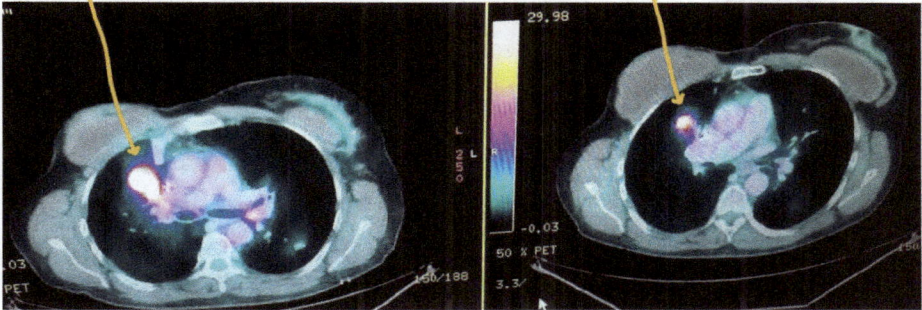

So what did you do?

I did Stereotactic Radiation Therapy on the tumor!

Did it help?

It bought me a few months. Enough time to take a vacation to Lake Powell with my kids, grandkids and my hubby.

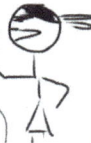

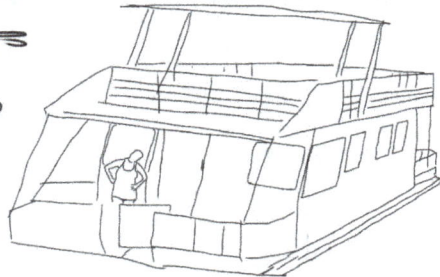

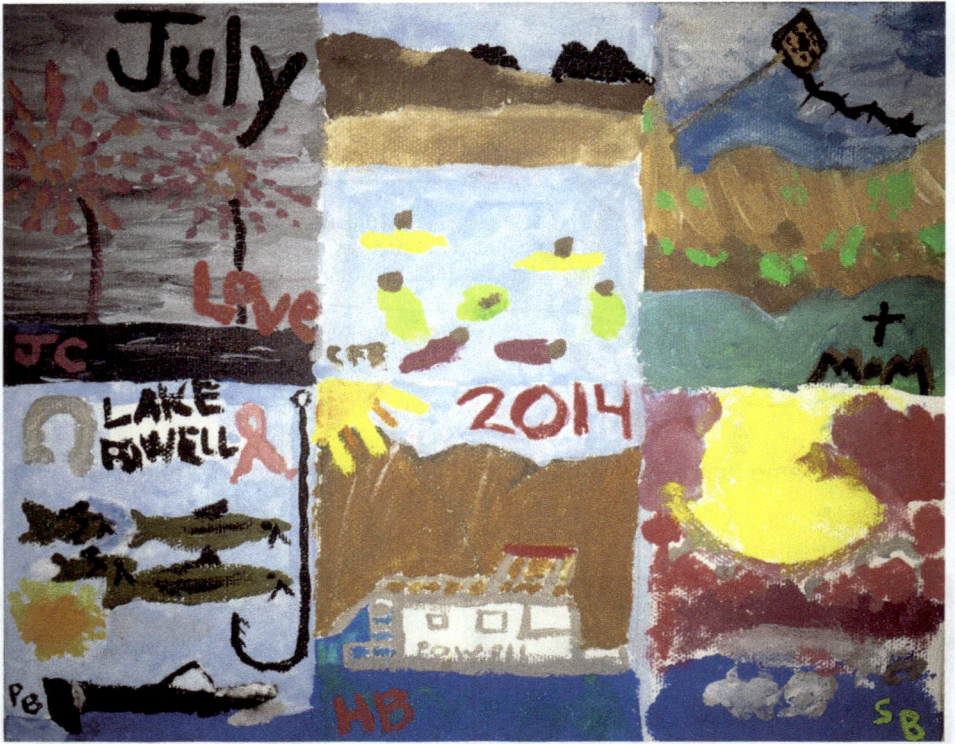

Neuropathy (at the mall)

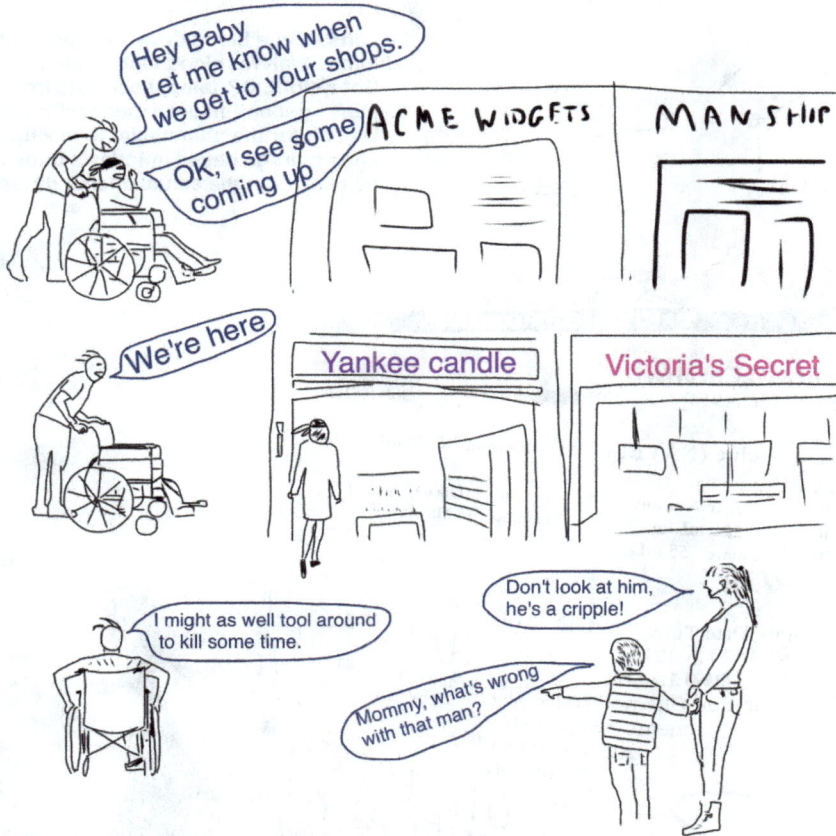

The side-effect of some chemo treatments is neuropathy. Neuropathy causes your hands and feet to go numb over time until you need to quit the chemo before it becomes permanent. Just walking can make your feet numb after just a few minutes.

Chemo Day Timeline

30 mins - Get a blood draw from phlebotomist.
60 mins - Wait for blood test results.
Get weight, BP, temp, heart rate from nurse.
60 mins - get anti-nausea meds infused while
waiting for the pharmacist to mix up the
chemo drugs based in today's body weight.
15-60 mins - get the actual chemo drugs infused.

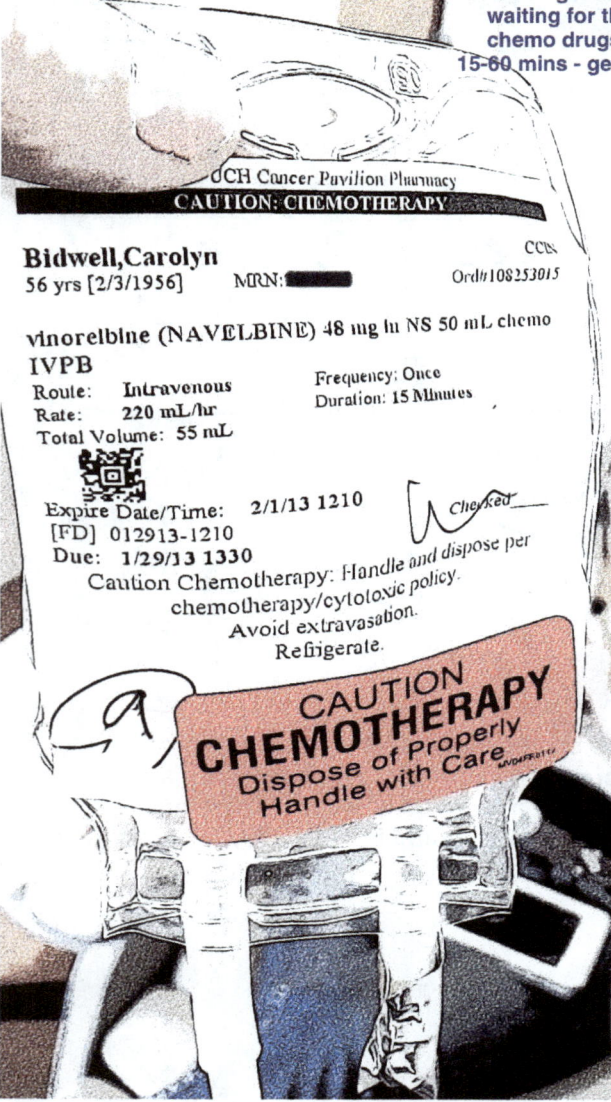

OCH Cancer Pavilion Pharmacy
CAUTION: CHEMOTHERAPY

Bidwell,Carolyn
56 yrs [2/3/1956]   MRN: Ord#108253015   CCN

vinorelbine (NAVELBINE) 48 mg in NS 50 mL chemo
IVPB
Route: Intravenous
Rate: 220 mL/hr
Total Volume: 55 mL

Frequency: Once
Duration: 15 Minutes

Expire Date/Time: 2/1/13 1210
[FD] 012913-1210
Due: 1/29/13 1330
Caution Chemotherapy: Handle and dispose per
chemotherapy/cytotoxic policy.
Avoid extravasation.
Refrigerate.

Checked

CAUTION
CHEMOTHERAPY
Dispose of Properly
Handle with Care

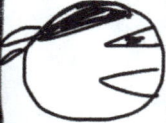

Actually the last step
is to have your husband
take you out for a nice
dinner on the way home,
or some shopping
as a treat.

It might just be the
hospital gift shop
if I'm feeling crappy

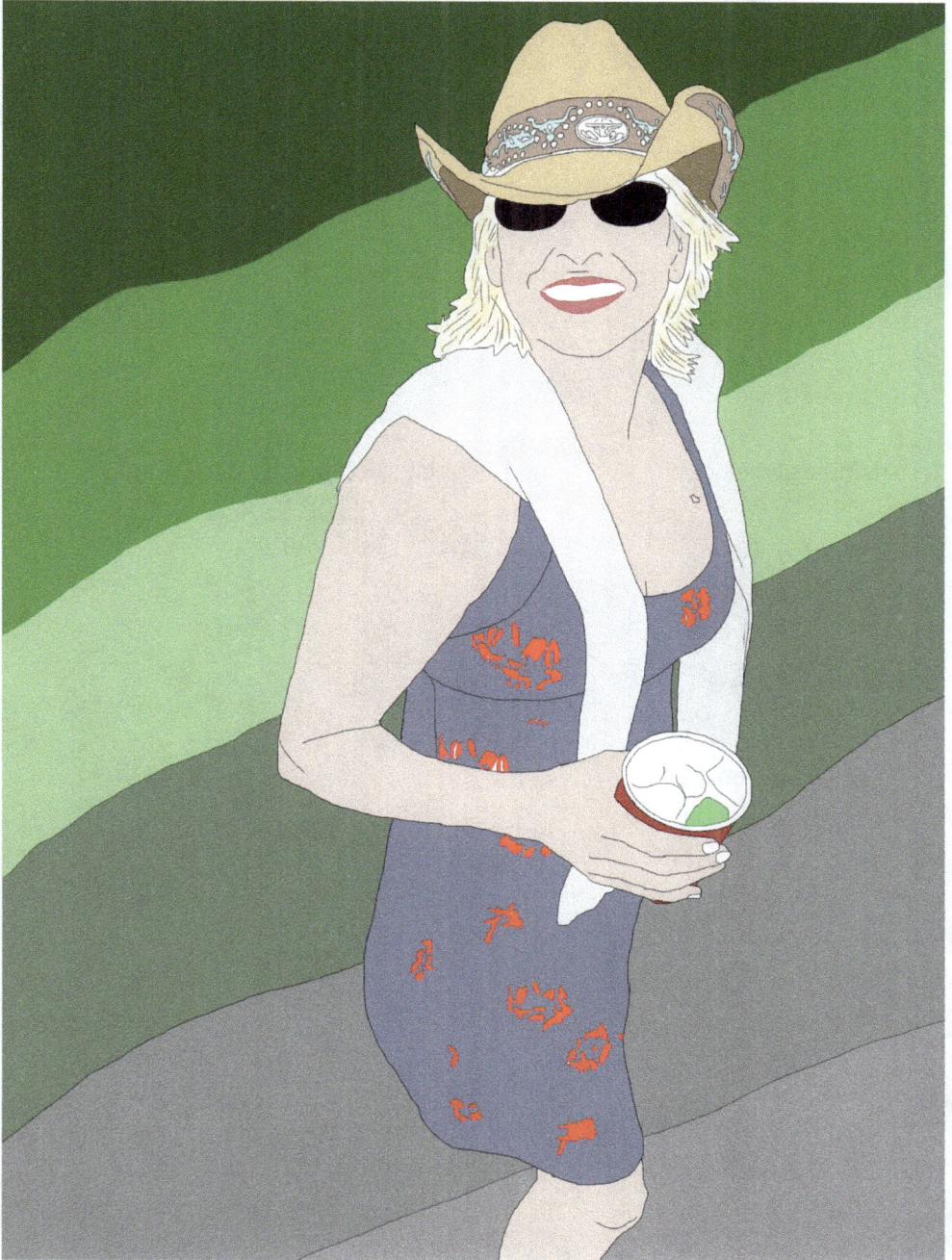

Cancer & Procrastination

November 30, 10:00 PM

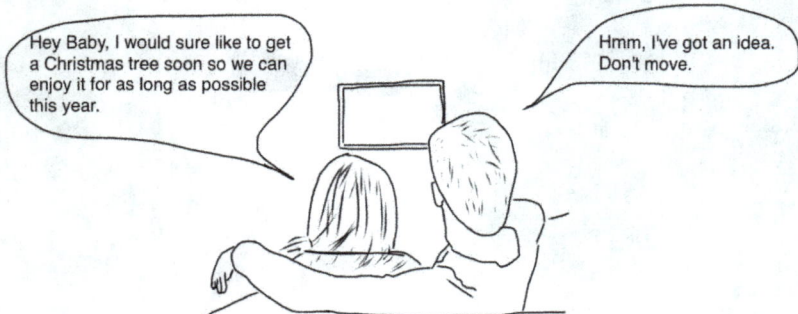

Minutes later...

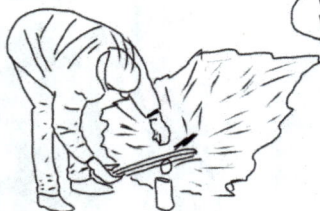

1 hour later

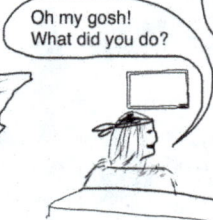

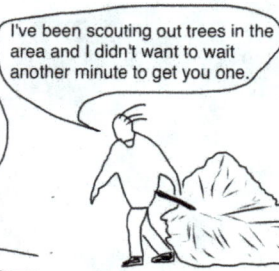

Late that evening

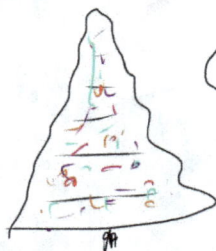

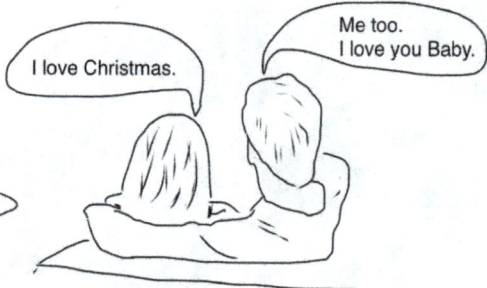

With cancer, even non-metastatic,
there is no time to lose for anything.

Scars

Cancer treatment is a lot like getting a tattoo.

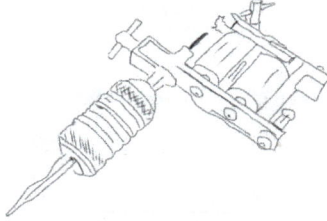

It hurts when you are getting it.
When done, you are scarred for life

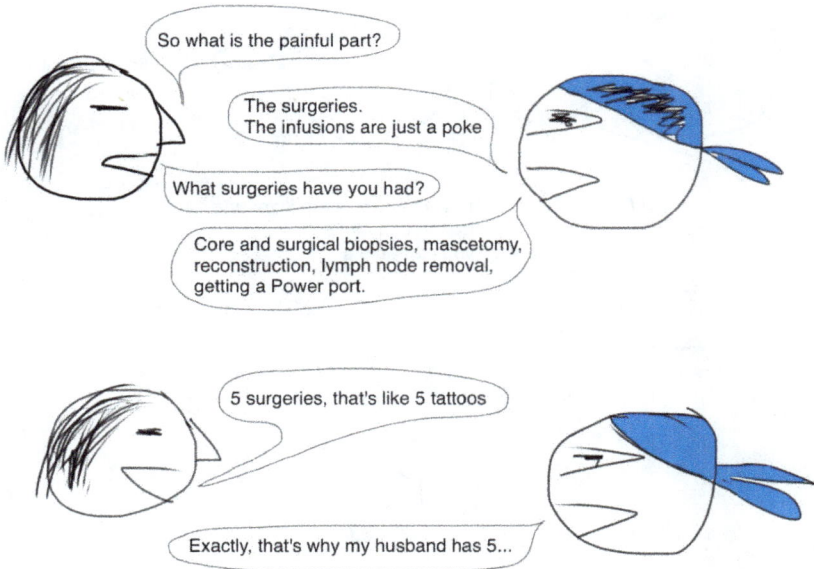

So what is the painful part?

The surgeries.
The infusions are just a poke

What surgeries have you had?

Core and surgical biopsies, mascetomy, reconstruction, lymph node removal, getting a Power port.

5 surgeries, that's like 5 tattoos

Exactly, that's why my husband has 5...

Chemo side-effects

All chemo drugs have a list of side-effects as long as your arm.
These are some common reactions for the drug Gemzar.
They also all have a long list of "Serious Reactions" that can be life
 threatening.

If you can handle these, the drugs can prolong or even save your
life depending on the cancer stage.
If not then you can try another drug with a different list of side-effects.

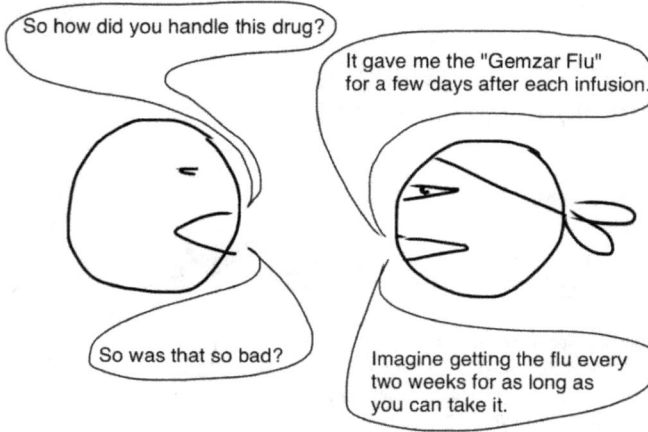

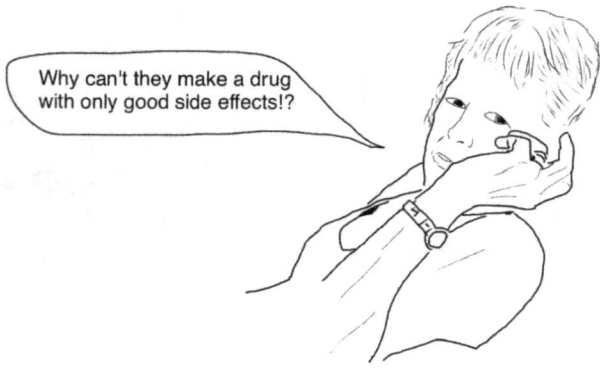

Common Reactions
- nausea
- vomiting
- anemia
- LFTs elevated
- neutropenia
- leukopenia
- pain
- fever
- hematuria
- proteinuria
- rash
- dyspnea
- constipation
- thrombocytopenia
- diarrhea
- hemorrhage
- infection
- alopecia
- stomatitis
- edema
- peripheral edema
- paresthesia
- flu syndrome
- somnolence

So how did you handle this drug?

It gave me the "Gemzar Flu" for a few days after each infusion.

So was that so bad?

Imagine getting the flu every two weeks for as long as you can take it.

Why can't they make a drug with only good side effects!?

Mastectomy & Reconstruction

When initially diagnosed with breast cancer, often a mastectomy is an excellent choice to remove the cancerous body part.

A round or two of chemo and/or radiation might be done to eradicate as much of the disease as possible before and after the mastectomy.

An expander is placed under the pectoral muscle during the mastectomy surgery. Several follow-up visits are needed to slowly fill up the expander to the desired cup size.

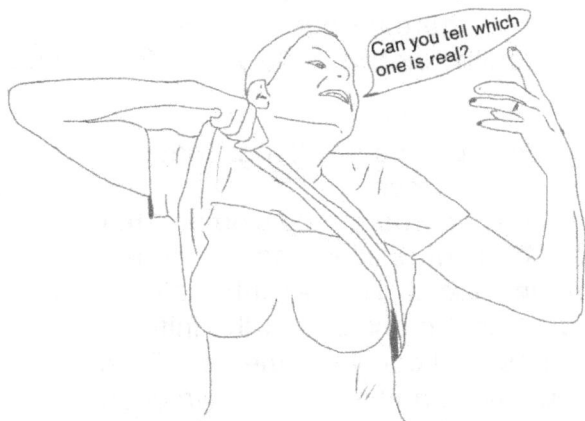

If just a unilateral (single breast) mastectomy, a breast implant may be put into the other breast so that they match.

6 months or so later, a final surgery is performed to replace the expander with an implant.

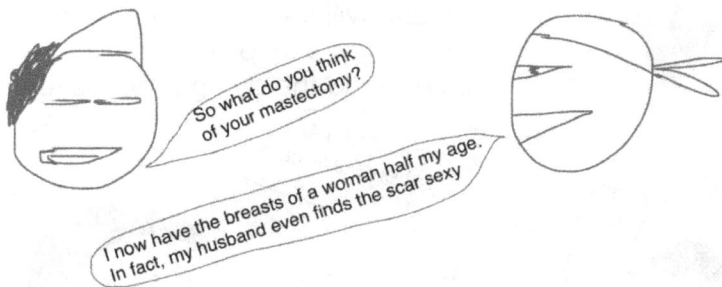

Surviving Metastatic Breast Cancer

A woman whose breast cancer has metastasized (Stage 4) lives knowing she can no longer be cured.

As her husband, no matter how much strength, knowledge or motivation I have, there is nothing I could do to save my wife. All I could do was be there for her and love her. Exercising and eating a healthy diet will help you to feel better, but will not cure you

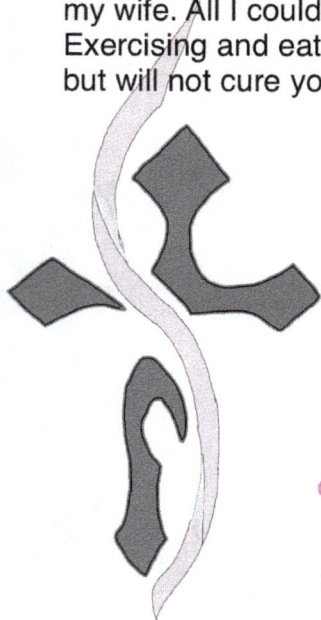

Carolyn did have two things that did save her however.
The first is modern medicine and her team of highly skilled doctors, especially her Oncologist. They kept her alive for 6 years and 4 months after the initial diagnosis. Those were the best 6 years of our lives, partly because we cherished our time together, but mostly because we were in love.
The second is God and Jesus.
Our faith will keep her soul alive for eternity, and that gave us peace.
It also made the dying process less scary.

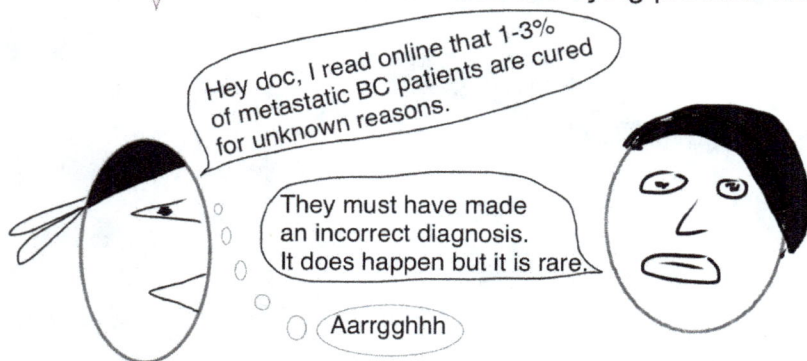

Hey doc, I read online that 1-3% of metastatic BC patients are cured for unknown reasons.

They must have made an incorrect diagnosis. It does happen but it is rare.

Aarrgghhh

Hospice & Palliative Care

When you start in-home hospice, you lose your insurance and are on Medicare, meaning you lose access to your doctors & your whole support network that you have built up.

It's not like a real hospice where there are doctors and nurses around the clock, in fact you won't see a doctor since they don't make house calls.

A better choice is palliative care. A nurse or social worker will visit you every week or two and give you advice. They will get you setup with a real hospice when it is needed. You continue with your insurance and doctors.

In a hospice, a doctor supervises infusing you with morphine, something that cannot be done at home where pills are the only option.

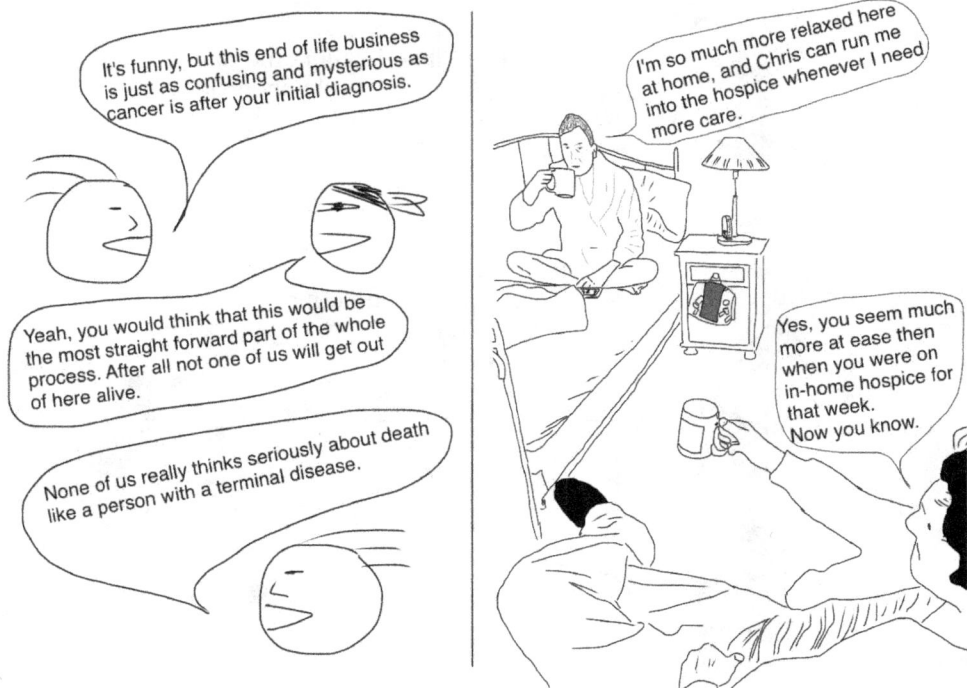

It's funny, but this end of life business is just as confusing and mysterious as cancer is after your initial diagnosis.

I'm so much more relaxed here at home, and Chris can run me into the hospice whenever I need more care.

Yeah, you would think that this would be the most straight forward part of the whole process. After all not one of us will get out of here alive.

Yes, you seem much more at ease then when you were on in-home hospice for that week. Now you know.

None of us really thinks seriously about death like a person with a terminal disease.

Cancer and falling

Whenever you go in to the doctors office, the hospital or the infusion center, there are a series of questions that they always ask you.
One of the big questions is "Have you fallen recently".
BTW, Carolyn never had to answer "Yes" to this question.

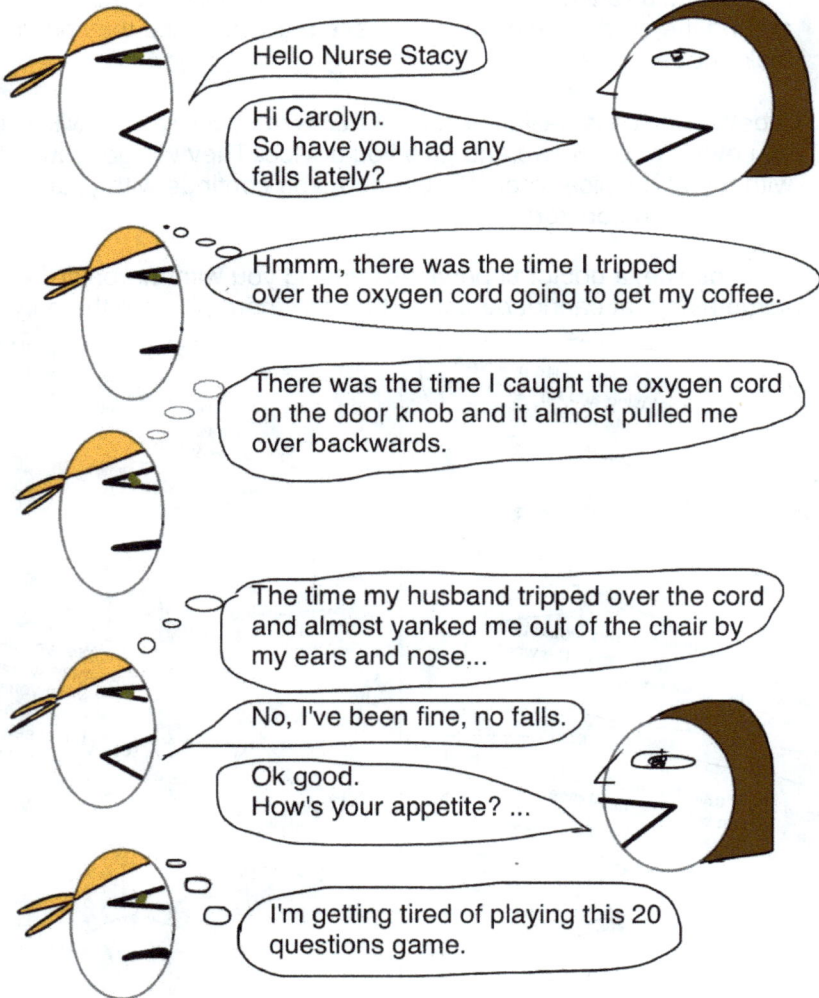

Hello Nurse Stacy

Hi Carolyn.
So have you had any falls lately?

Hmmm, there was the time I tripped over the oxygen cord going to get my coffee.

There was the time I caught the oxygen cord on the door knob and it almost pulled me over backwards.

The time my husband tripped over the cord and almost yanked me out of the chair by my ears and nose...

No, I've been fine, no falls.

Ok good.
How's your appetite? ...

I'm getting tired of playing this 20 questions game.

Love & cancer

Strictly speaking, this is is not about cancer,
but it does show that love transcends everything,
including that bitch cancer.
These are some poems & quotes from Carolyn over the years.

(2003) The light in you has exposed the love I have to give.
This love, buried for a lifetime.
Can it be? True love at last!
Thank you Chris. My love.
The light in you reveals a man of great worth.
Knowing you, how could I live again without you?
Be with me Chris forever.

(2004) "You fill my heart today with gladness.
I love you - all of you, inside and out. The creation itself makes
me think of you. Everything God thought of and made thrills
me because he included you, then he gave you to me. Wow!
You have my heart, soul, body and mind and know I love you."

(2007) "I love you and you always make me smile."

(2010) "How cool to live and sleep with your best friend.
The one who loves you, and says it constantly and listens and
responds to your every emotional or intellectual thought and idea.
But guess what, It took till I was 47 to find him. Never give up!!!"

(2012) "I just wanted to grow old with you".
(2012) "Thank you for your love you give me.
Because of you, my life is wonderful every day."

(2014) "I could never love anyone as much as I love you.
Thank you for showing me - teaching me real love like I've never
known before. May we have much more time together to be in love
and to share our love."

This image of Carolyn's tattoo has special meaning since it symbolizes several things.

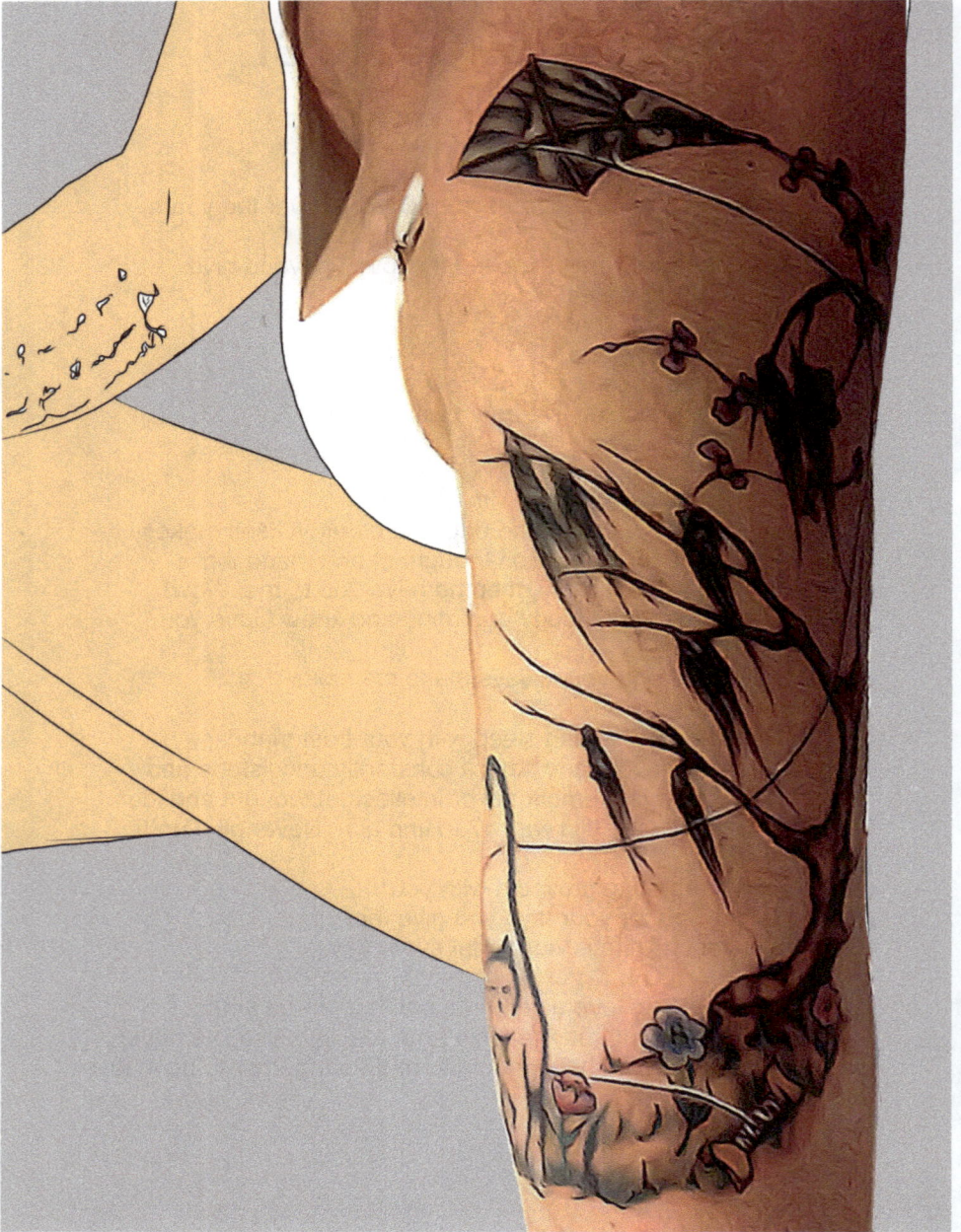

Carolyn had wanted a tattoo for a while and she ended up getting her first one on her year of being cancer-free. No, it was not a pink cancer ribbon tramp stamp, but a cross with a cancer ribbon through it on her right shoulder blade (not long afterwards, her daughter Hailey and I both got the same matching tattoos as Carolyn). It was fortuitous since she was diagnosed with Metastatic cancer just three weeks later. After that she really did not want to get any other tattoos since her time was now limited and what's the point of getting a new tattoo if you won't be around to wear it and enjoy showing it off. This new attitude also applied to clothes, cars, electronics and especially jewelry, partly because she was a stickler for not wasting money, but mostly since she had a fatalistic attitude towards life since the terminal cancer diagnosis. She had mentioned to me before that she had always wanted a diamond engagement ring since she had never had one. To help change her mindset, at Christmas that year I got her a very nice diamond ring. She realized that we all have limited time on earth, so why deprive yourself of things that you would enjoy if you did not have cancer. As it turned out she did get to wear that ring for almost 4 years. She also got several other tattoos and would not worry about how long she would wear them, as she was getting more comfortable with her terminal disease, which is really what metastatic cancer is. All of her tattoos are scattered throughout this book. In fact she got her last tattoo, which is in the picture above, just 10 months before she died.

The image also shows how comfortable she was with her body. She was aware of the toll that cancer and the chemotherapy took. Things like surgery scars, ports, a mastectomy, steroid body changes, thin or no hair and dry skin that makes you look older, but there is not much you can do about it. I told her that all the things that she went through for her entire life shaped her and made her the woman that I loved. Cancer was just giving her more character and was adding to her beauty. I really wanted to be with her even more as she was going through all the treatments. She would get concerned about how she looked and it helped to tell her the truth, "you look beautiful baby".

In the winter when it is cold and blowing outside we would keep the house as warm as we could. Sometimes we would keep it at 75 or even 80 degrees downstairs where the house is really well insulated and the pellet stove really cranks out the heat. Our mountain house has a real cottage feel and we would kid each other about being at the beach in the mountains, all we were lacking were the sand and sea outside our door. When she peeled off her clothes to a "wife beater" or tank top, then I knew that we were successful. Life is too short to be freezing in a sweater inside your house for the winter and this image really shows that too!

Bald From Chemo

Not all chemo treatments will cause you to lose your hair, but most target fast growing cells and that includes hair.

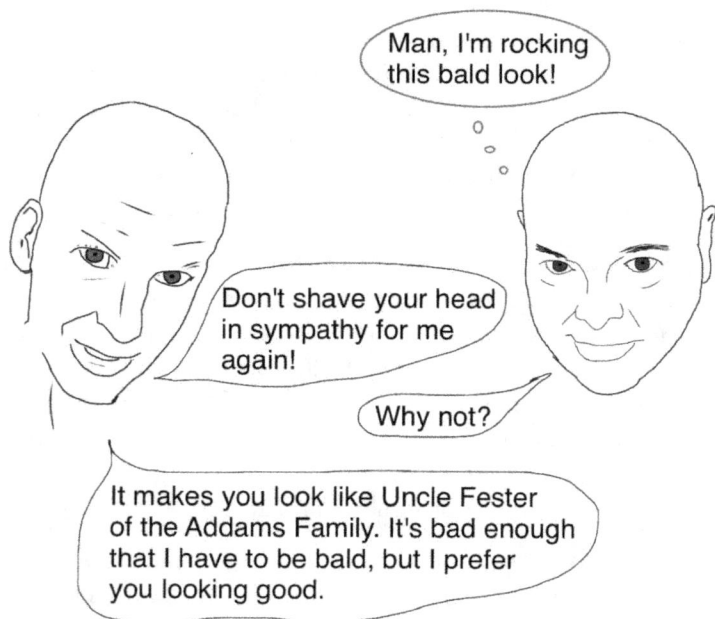

Man, I'm rocking this bald look!

Don't shave your head in sympathy for me again!

Why not?

It makes you look like Uncle Fester of the Addams Family. It's bad enough that I have to be bald, but I prefer you looking good.

Tip - Don't shave you're head, but trim to stubble. This gives your scarves, Buffs, wigs and head coverings something to grab onto.
The stubble is also less likely to fall out than longer hair.

Living In the Moment

Riding is great. It's an adventure every time and it is not exhausting like climbing a 14er.

Biking is something exciting that we could do and be totally together. Communication is mostly by touch, so it is also intimate.

Your mind wanders, especially on long trips. She would not think about cancer and I would not think about work. We would both have epiphanies and could hardly wait till he next stop to tell each other about them.

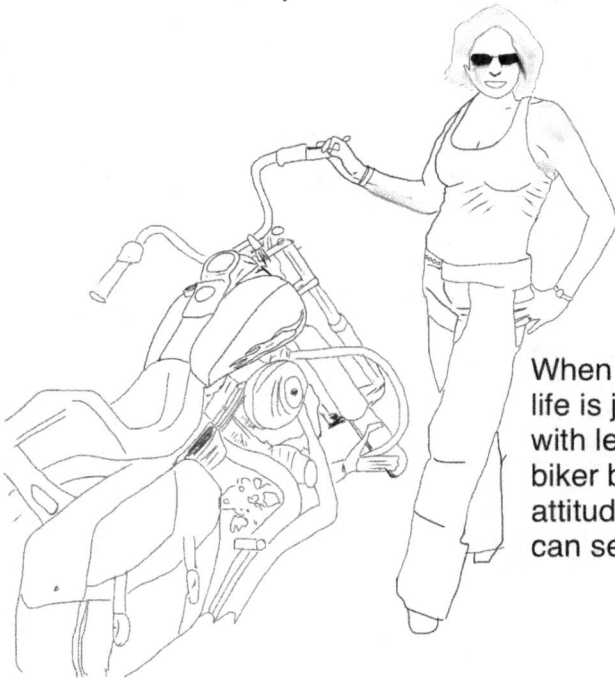

When biking you are living totally in the moment.

When not on the bike, life is just a little different with leathers, bandanas, biker boots and a little attitude. Just like you can see on her face here.

Chemo & Menopause

Chemo will reduce the amount of hormones that a woman's body produces, often throwing you into early menopause.

Carolyn was at the normal age for menopause so it came on quickly with the chemo, but it can happen to women in their 30s and 40s also.

One main side effect is hot flashes that can come on at any time.

Typically after a hot flash, you get cold since your sweat cools off and chills you. It's an almost impossible task to keep the house cool enough and hot enough to stay comfortable.

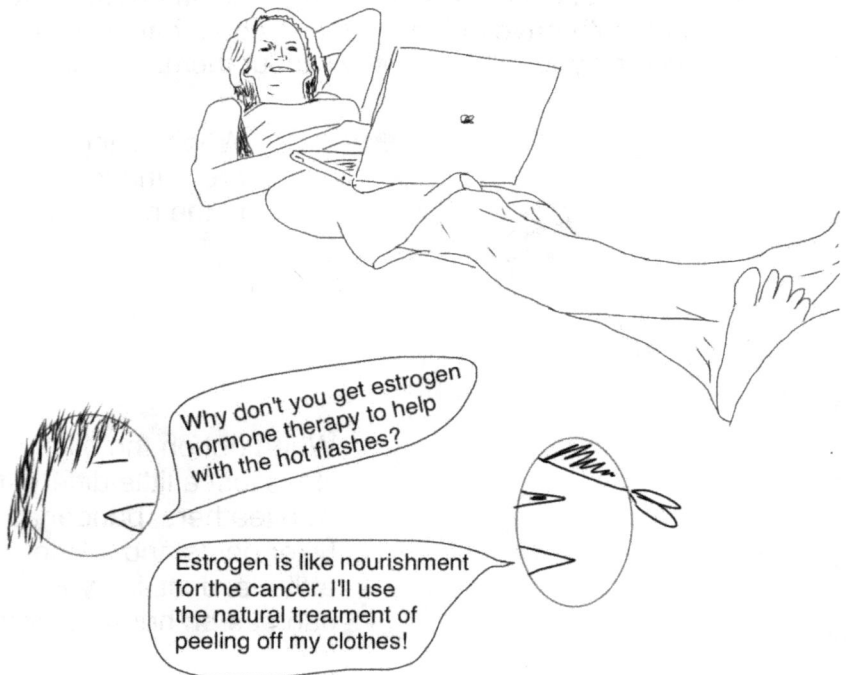

Why don't you get estrogen hormone therapy to help with the hot flashes?

Estrogen is like nourishment for the cancer. I'll use the natural treatment of peeling off my clothes!

Grandkids and Memory

Carolyn was always worried that her grandkids would not remember her.

Somehow I don't think that that should be a worry.

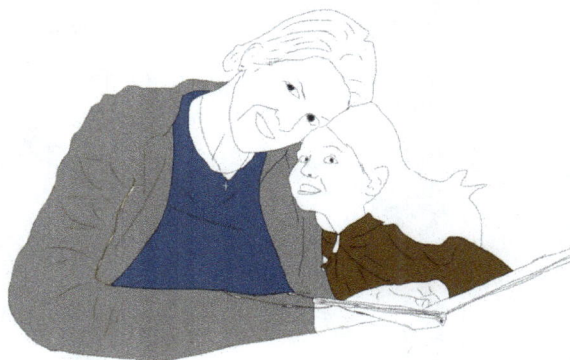

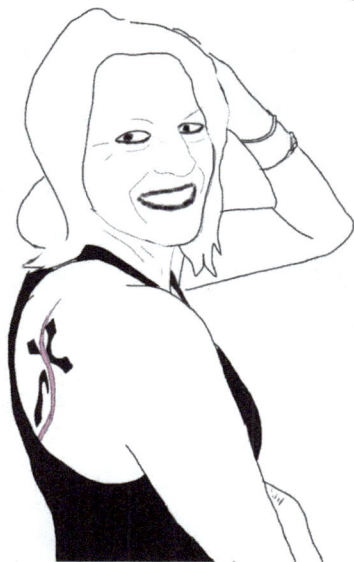

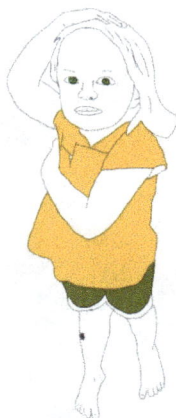

Even if their memory of her fades over time, they will be mimicking her behavior forever.

Road trips

Sometimes when you need a break from the routine nothing beats a road trip.

On our last road trip to the Grand Canyon, Disneyland and Santa Monica, we just talked the entire trip, except once when Carolyn was getting into driving the TT fast and wanted some loud music.

I'm always envious of how comfortable women can be in the car with just a little dress.

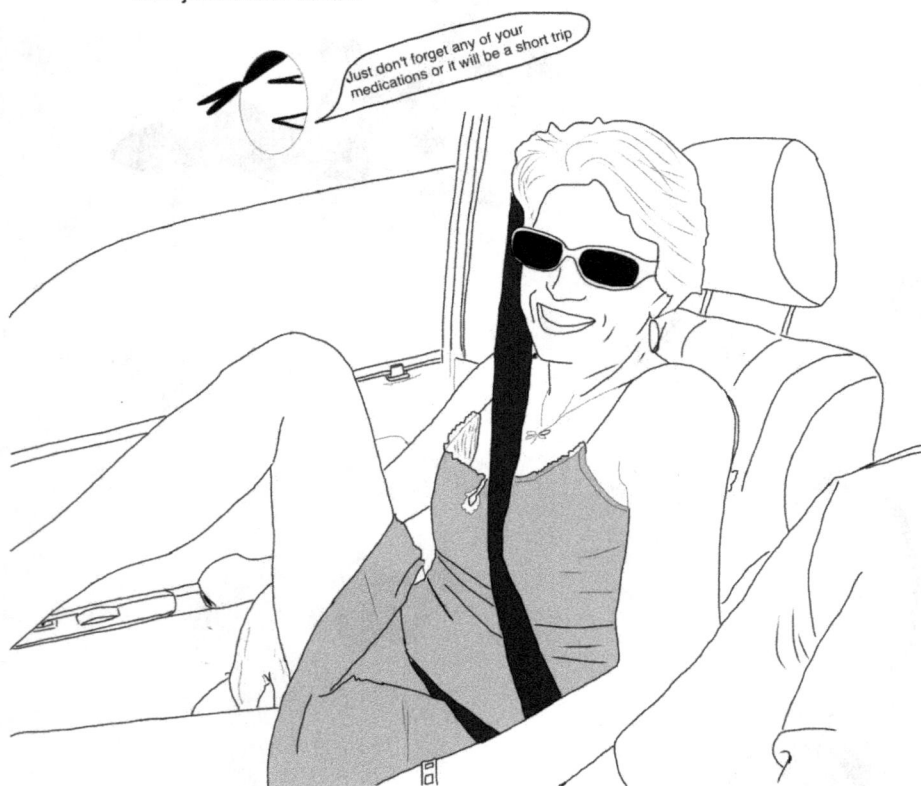

The First Week

In many ways the first week after your initial diagnosis is the hardest. You are still reeling from the fact that you have cancer. The treatment, the tests, the doctors, the machines and equipment are all new. You are embarking on a journey into the unknown, and you could die.

This is a glimpse into our first week.

Tue   I rushed home from a business trip to be with Carolyn. We hugged and talked about our feelings, which was mostly numbness. I assured her that we would get through this together and that I loved her more than ever.

Wed   We went to Boulder and got the biopsy reports, mammogram & ultrasound films. We grabbed lunch and comforted each other. After lunch we had her 1st MRI scan which suprised me with the noise.

Thur   We went back to Boulder Hospital and had a pet scan that lasted for a couple hours. Instead of lunch, we just sat on a bench in a hallway and I had my arm around her and we snuggled tight. We then got a CD of all the scans since we were switching care to the Anschutz Cancer Center at University Hospital. On the drive home Carolyn talked about how scared she was of this breast cancer and it really made me feel protective of her.

Fri, Sat, Sun   Over the weekend we barely left each other's side since she was having a hard time dealing with the crushing weight of the reality of the cancer. I did take her to Golden to watch me go kayaking, but that was probably more of an escape for me.

Mon   We got the results of the PET scan that showed no cancer elsewhere in her body! That was some measure of relief.

Tue   We met with the new Oncologist, Radiologist and med students. We had so many questions that I used my laptop to make notes of everything. Downstairs at the pharmacy we filled prescriptions for Effexor, Percocet and Xanex (for pain and anxiety). We returned a bit later to get 6 painful core biopsies on her right breast to get the "source of the cancer". This is necessary to determine the course of the chemo treatments.

People's Initial Reactions

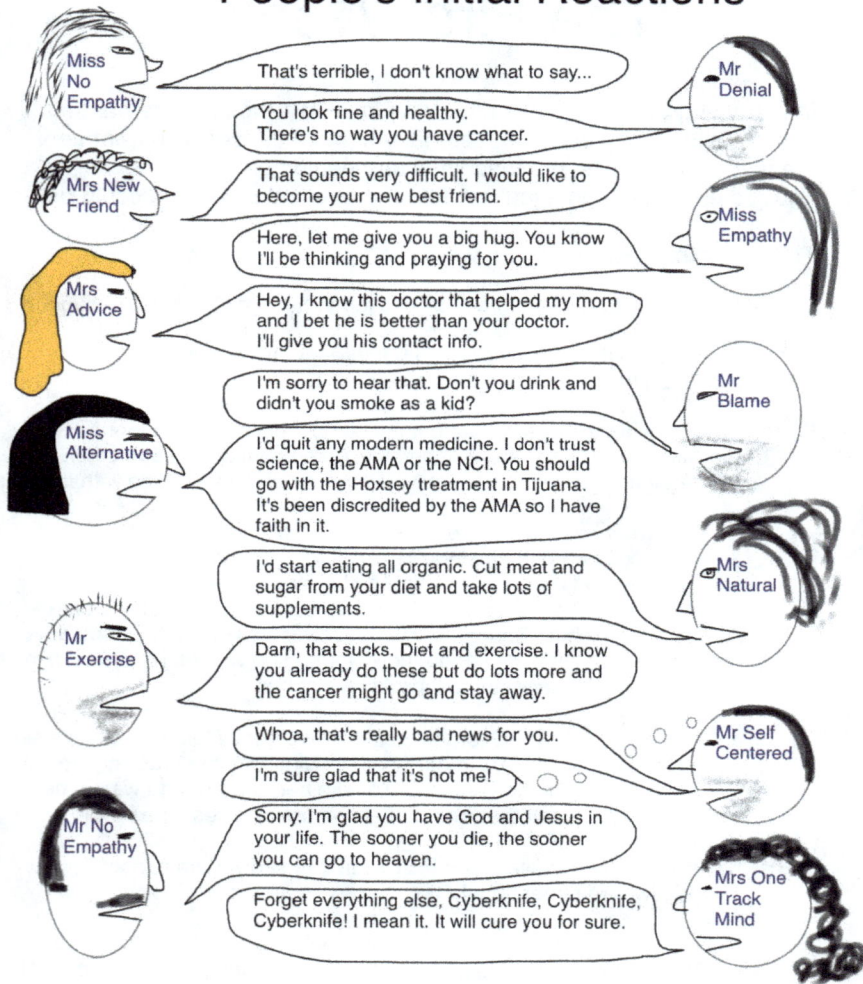

Miss No Empathy

That's terrible, I don't know what to say...

Mr Denial

You look fine and healthy.
There's no way you have cancer.

Mrs New Friend

That sounds very difficult. I would like to become your new best friend.

Miss Empathy

Here, let me give you a big hug. You know I'll be thinking and praying for you.

Mrs Advice

Hey, I know this doctor that helped my mom and I bet he is better than your doctor. I'll give you his contact info.

I'm sorry to hear that. Don't you drink and didn't you smoke as a kid?

Mr Blame

Miss Alternative

I'd quit any modern medicine. I don't trust science, the AMA or the NCI. You should go with the Hoxsey treatment in Tijuana. It's been discredited by the AMA so I have faith in it.

I'd start eating all organic. Cut meat and sugar from your diet and take lots of supplements.

Mrs Natural

Mr Exercise

Darn, that sucks. Diet and exercise. I know you already do these but do lots more and the cancer might go and stay away.

Whoa, that's really bad news for you.

Mr Self Centered

I'm sure glad that it's not me!

Mr No Empathy

Sorry. I'm glad you have God and Jesus in your life. The sooner you die, the sooner you can go to heaven.

Forget everything else, Cyberknife, Cyberknife, Cyberknife! I mean it. It will cure you for sure.

Mrs One Track Mind

Cats & Ports

Cats are a constant source of comfort and companionship.
She liked males that would get more attached to her.
I like them for their awesome mousing abilities.
There was always a cat or two following her around or on her side of the bed.
In her last few weeks, they barely left her side.

Here she is "torturing" them under the covers.

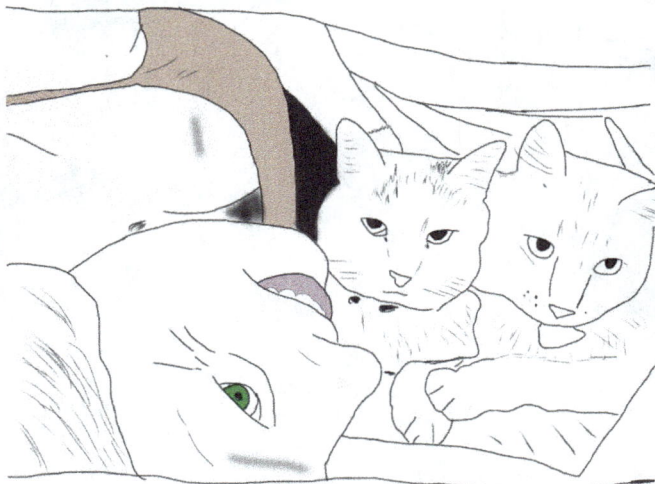

You can see the infusion port scar on her breast. They are easily recognized on women who have had chemo. I had a nice talk with a woman cutting my hair that I would not have known was a BC survivor if not for the scar.

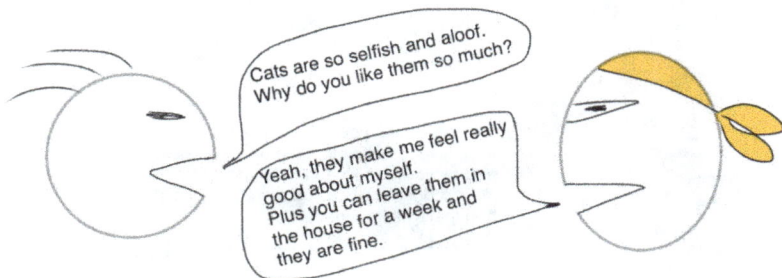

Cats are so selfish and aloof. Why do you like them so much?

Yeah, they make me feel really good about myself. Plus you can leave them in the house for a week and they are fine.

Life Accelerated

One problem with chemo therapy, is that it is like normal life, but accelerated.

The chemo will dry out your skin and thin out your hair (if you have any) losing its luster and body, making you look older than you are.

It will sap your energy and endurance, making you feel older than you really are.

If the cancer has metastasized (spread from the breast and hence terminal) then you have just a few years left like an elderly person.

You will want to take all those trips that most people put off till retirement.

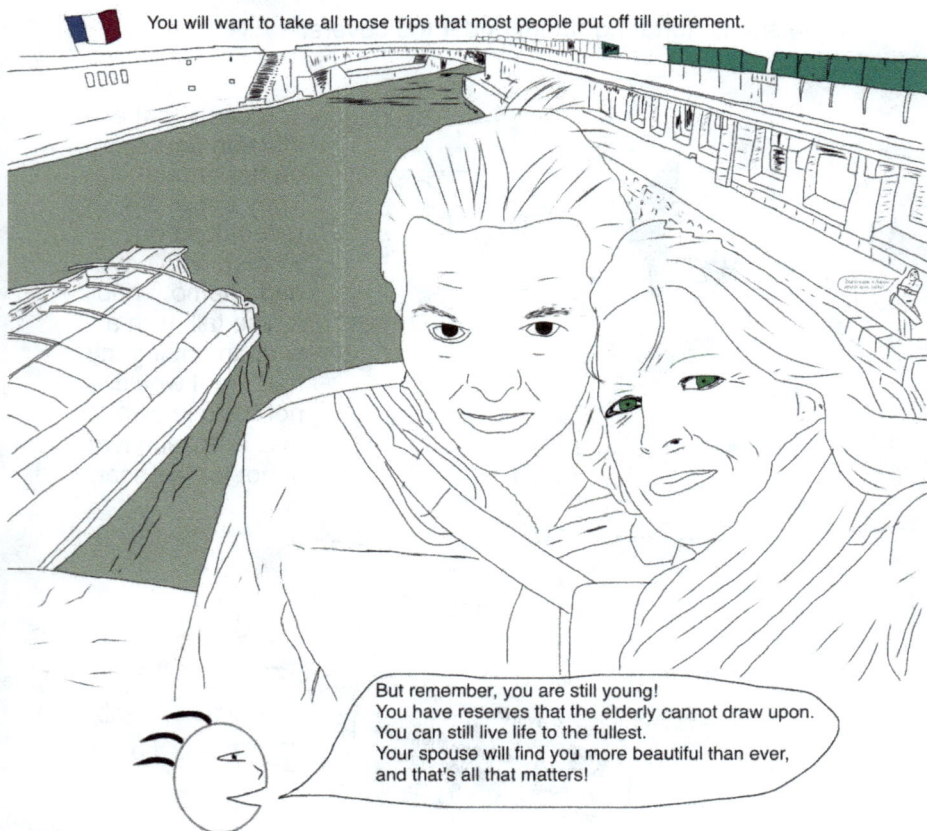

But remember, you are still young!
You have reserves that the elderly cannot draw upon.
You can still live life to the fullest.
Your spouse will find you more beautiful than ever,
and that's all that matters!

Traveling Without a Plan

Sometimes you feel like hitting as many sights as possible, and sometimes you feel like just finding a coffee shop and have a low-energy day.

We call it being locals for a day

Often times those "being local" days would be the most memorable part of the trip. It also eliminates the stress of having an immutable schedule.

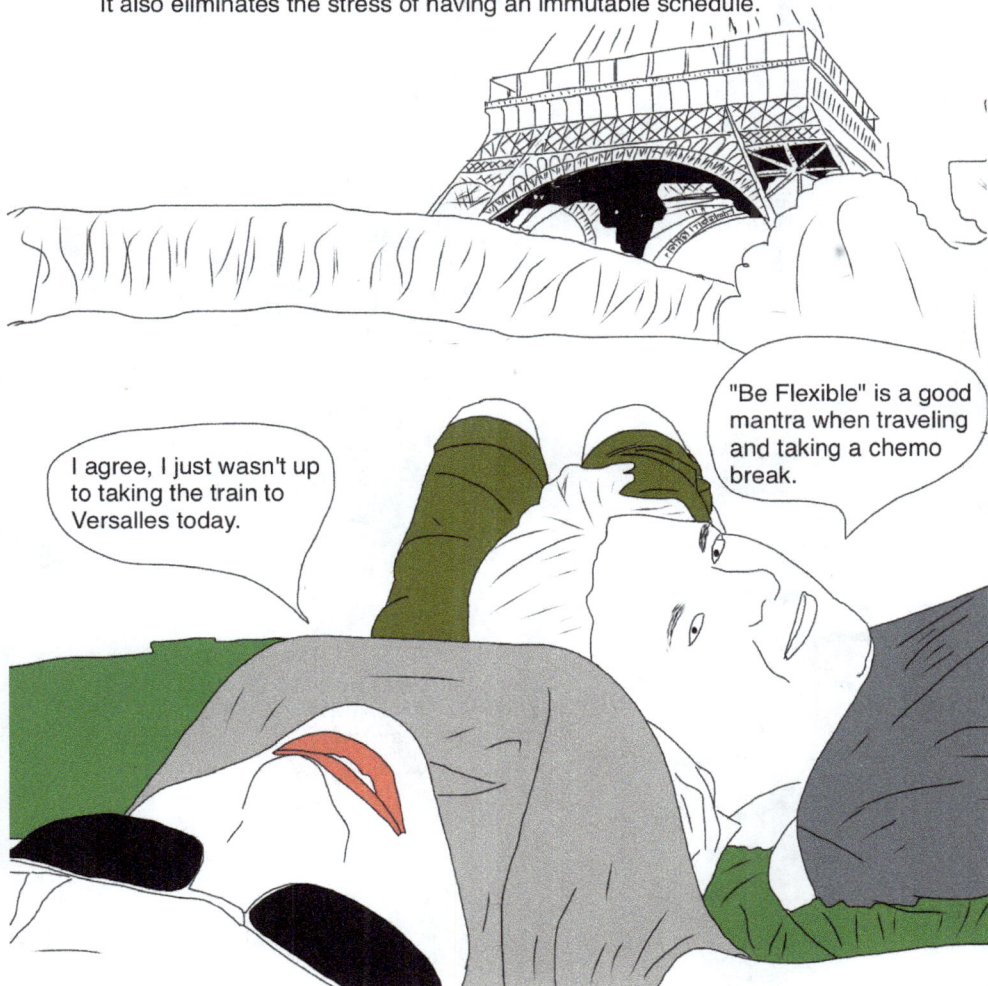

"Be Flexible" is a good mantra when traveling and taking a chemo break.

I agree, I just wasn't up to taking the train to Versalles today.

Wonderfully Mad

Some Chemos will wreak havoc on your emotions. It can cause you to get mad, sad, anxious, scared or depressed when you normally would not.

Just go with the flow. It's not her, it's the marvelous evil brew coursing through her veins that is fighting for her life!

Here she is miffed at me for pulling us off the Tube platform during rush hour and going up to a pub to kill an hour sipping on pints.

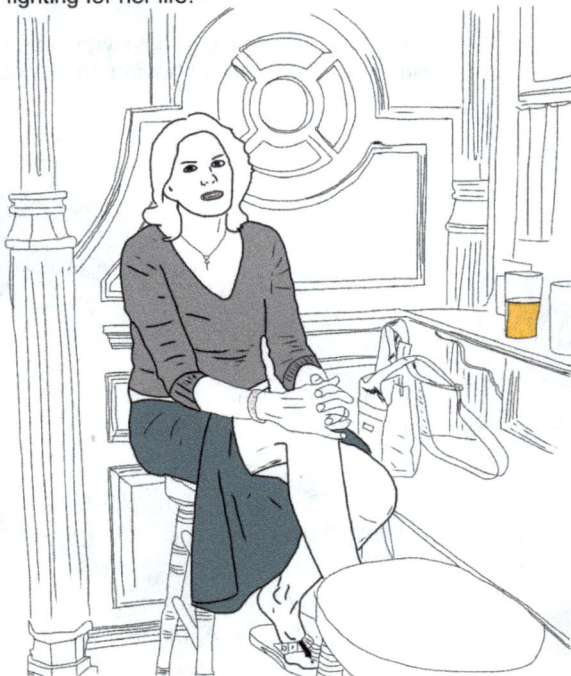

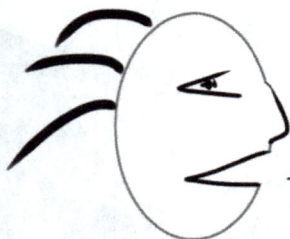

Women are beautiful when they smile, but they are stunning when they flash those angry eyes at you.

The MRI Experience

People get worried, even scared about having an MRI scan but it is really just a fear of the unknown.
This Insight will help to remove that fear.

The MRI machine mostly just makes a lot of noise.
To get an idea download and play The Rockafeller Skank by Fatboy Slim.
Put on your headphones and crank it up and listen to the whole song.
It will grow on you! See! It's not so bad.
And now you have a cool new rap/techno song in your music library.
I would hum this song on the way home after Carolyn had an MRI.

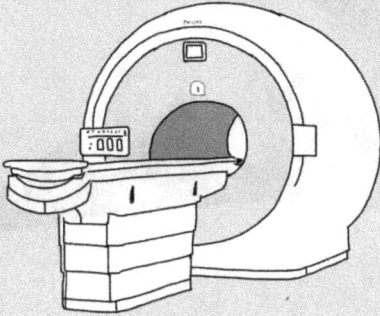

The machine itself is big and friendly looking, like a big egg. It is even open on both ends.

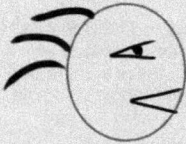

For sure go into the MRI room with your spouse during a scan, otherwise how can you both have a shared experience.

If you are claustrophobic, well nothing is even touching you.
It is nothing like crawling in a cave. Think of it as being in the womb of this huge machine that is desperately trying to save you!

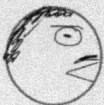

What about Praise You? That's a better song.

It's not about the song, it's about the experience.

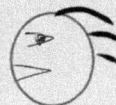

Mets Babes

A big part of your support network are those women who are going through exactly what you are going through. An excellent resource are the online support groups that are organized as chat rooms and all the members are women with cancer.

Carolyn started with the Crazy Sexy women and that was perfect when she was initially on chemo and was hoping for a cure. These women are positive almost to a fault about beating cancer and are into eating healthy.

When her cancer came back and it had metastasized (now terminal) she needed a more specialized support group.
That's when she became very active in the metastatic cancer women group on Facebook. They would chat for hours about reactions to chemo, side-effects of drugs, how the disease is spreading, enjoying life, end of life issues and spiritual support.

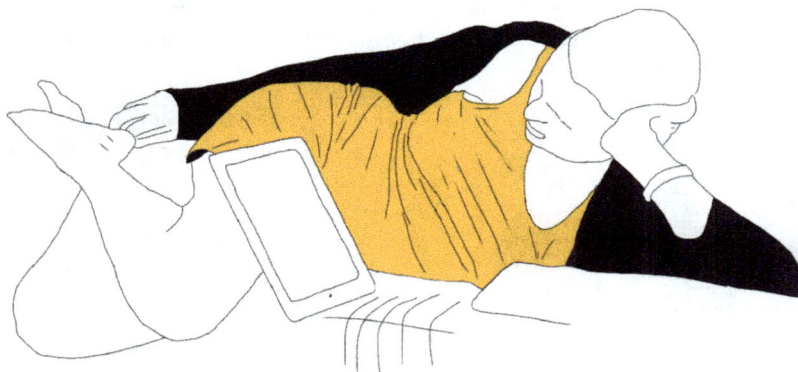

There are also specialized splinter groups such as "Stage 4 TNBC Sisters" for women with triple negative breast cancer (no ER, PR or HR tumor receptors) which is what Carolyn had. She became good friends with a number of these women and even got together with a few of them. It was always hard when her friends would die, but that's the reality of life.

When Carolyn died I got a nice bereavement card with the names of 82 women in her Mets Babes support group, that's how extensive her network was!

Relaxing Amongst the Chaos

Some people can just naturally relax in the chaos that surrounds them. Others might need a little help to mentally handle the disorder so they can enjoy the moment. Most of us need a little assistance and women with cancer need more than the rest of us.

Going to a quiet place to relax is often best.
A gin & tonic is a good choice to relax with. The chemotherapy never ruined the taste of this drink for her.
Xanex helps you to relax, but Carolyn only used it for a good nights sleep.
Some of the "Mets Babes" use Ativan. They refer to it as Ativantastic!

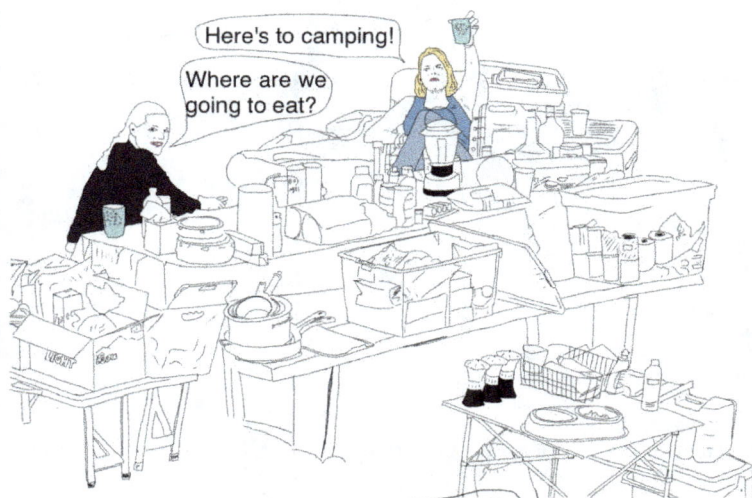

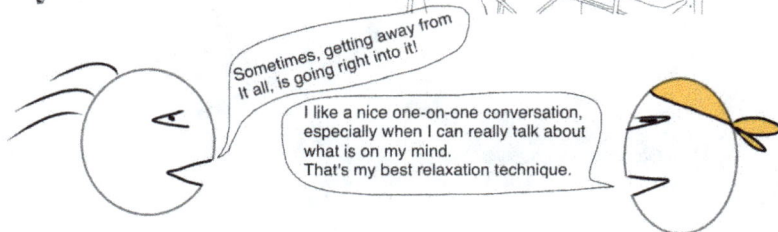

Here's to camping!

Where are we going to eat?

Sometimes, getting away from it all, is going right into it!

I like a nice one-on-one conversation, especially when I can really talk about what is on my mind.
That's my best relaxation technique.

Gardening

Creative activities that you enjoy and are relaxing are an excellent way to live in the moment and enjoy life.
Flower gardening is especially good. It gets you outside and in touch with nature, and the results are pretty immediate.

The chemo effects your taste, making foods you like start tasting bad, but the flowers always smell fragrant and wonderful.

Here Carolyn is getting a double shot of good smells from the purple Iris and the freshly ground Guatemalan coffee.

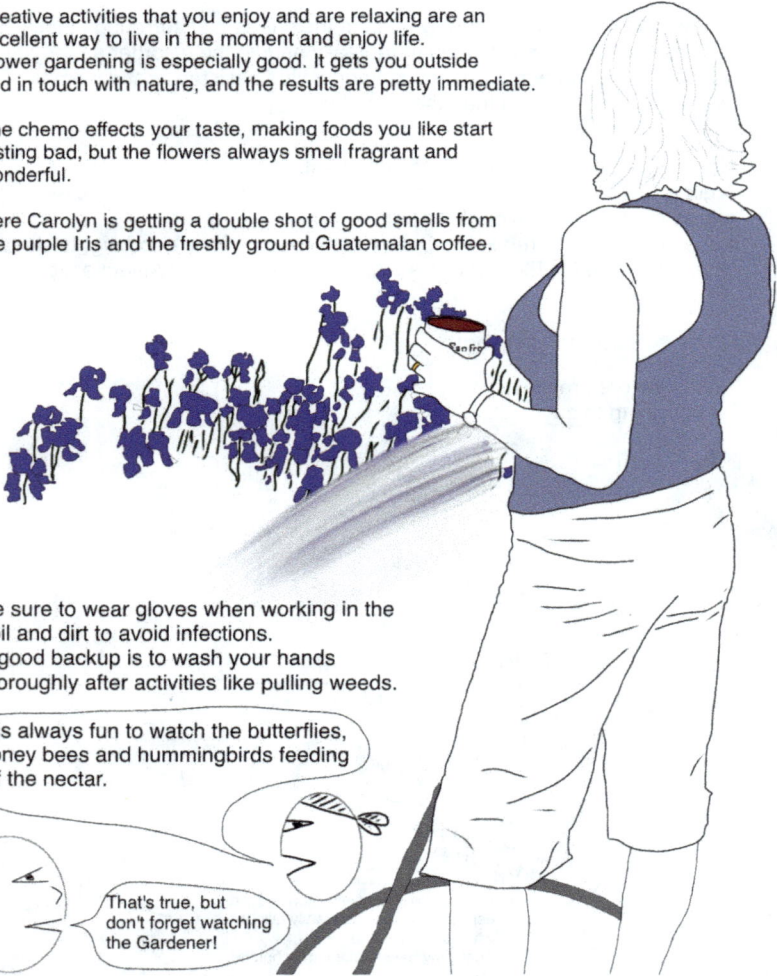

Be sure to wear gloves when working in the soil and dirt to avoid infections.
A good backup is to wash your hands thoroughly after activities like pulling weeds.

It is always fun to watch the butterflies, honey bees and hummingbirds feeding off the nectar.

That's true, but don't forget watching the Gardener!

TV Habits

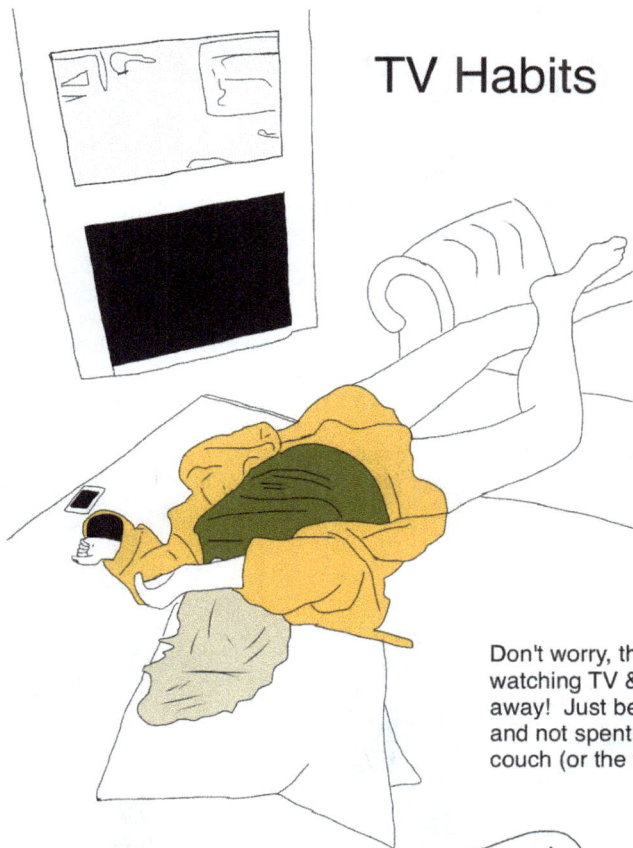

Rather than waiting for a season of a show to come out on Netflix, we changed to watching them as they aired.
Who knew if she would be around by the time they were available on disc.

We were disappointed that she could not finish Mad Men (1/2 season left) and Downton Abbey (missed final season).

Don't worry, there is no link between watching TV & breast cancer so watch away! Just be sure to keep active and not spent too much time on the couch (or the floor).

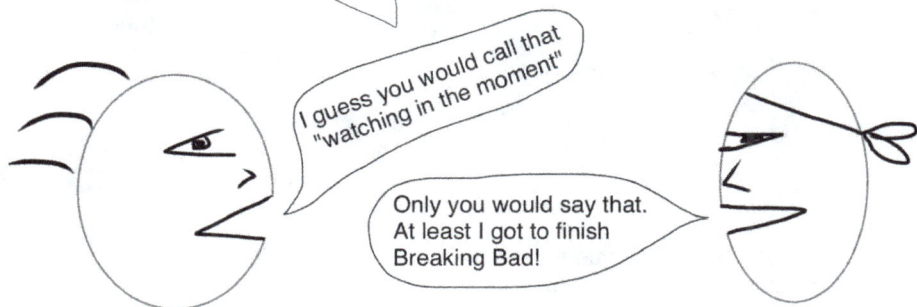

I guess you would call that "watching in the moment"

Only you would say that. At least I got to finish Breaking Bad!

Camping

It's always good to get away from the day to day of everyday life and what better way to do that than going camping.
When camping with cancer and chemo, the main idea is to "ease it" rather than "roughing it".

The easiest way to do that is with a camper.
Then you are sleeping in a comfy warm bed and you have a kitchen to make morning coffee in comfort. Camping can be pretty spur of the moment depending on where you want to go.

If you are not feeling well sometimes, the camper is your little escape pod while the others are out fishing or pitching horseshoes or just sitting around the campfire.

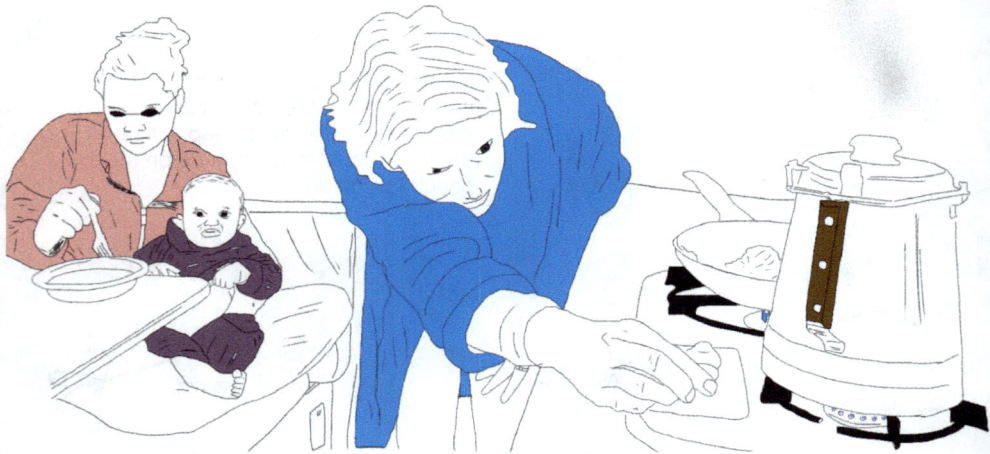

It's important to continue to do those things that you love and not cut them out of your life. You just might want your husband to do most of the packing and unpacking now, even if that is something that you enjoy, just so you don't get worn out.
He will be happy to do it since he will be going camping!

Working Out

Exercise is an important part of your lifestyle, especially when you are on chemo. Carolyn's favorite was lifting weights, either at the gym or at home.

We usually went on hikes for aerobic exercise. Later as Carolyn developed lung mets (the breast cancer metastasized to her lungs), the hikes turned into walks.

On some chemo treatments the neuropathy in her feet prevented long walks and she would concentrate on weight lifting.

BENEFITS
Lessen the risk of osteoporosis
Help keep a healthy weight
Lessen fatigue
Improve your balance
Keep your body toned
It makes you feel good (endorphins)

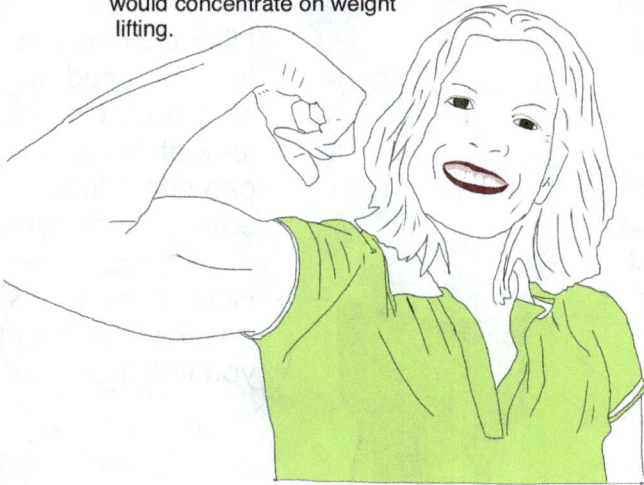

Be sure to drink plenty of water to avoid dehydration!

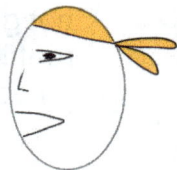

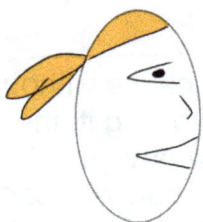

Hey, do you want to go workout now?

Ummm, I don't know. Perhaps later.

WHAT!? You are supposed to be encouraging me, not the other way around!

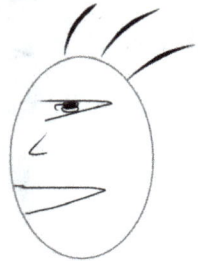

Dressing Up

Dressing up, whether going to a wedding, going to chemo or going to the mall can make you feel so good about yourself.

It shows your friends and loved ones that you have not given up and reaffirms the same for yourself.

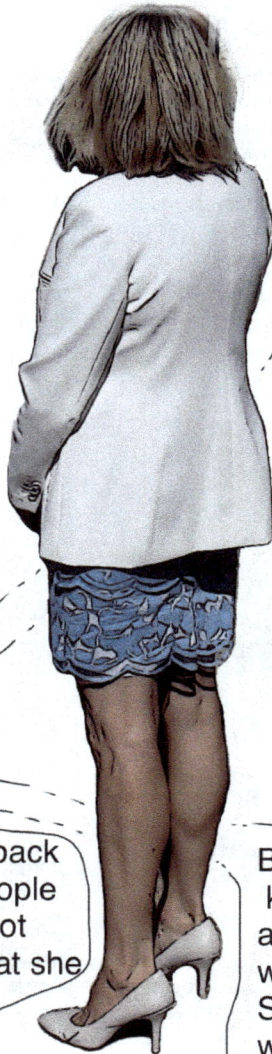

I like it when she is all dressed up and other women look at her and I can see a little envy in their eyes.

How could it possibly be that you like that!

The drawback is that people often do not believe that she is sick.

Because without knowing it, they are envious of a woman with cancer. She is just another woman.

Photography

Taking photos is a creative process that can also be very artistic. It can be landscapes, people, abstract expressions with manipulation, pets, kids, or whatever interests you.

Carolyn had a real knack for getting a great shot. We were in Barcelona and walked all around Antoni Gaudí's Sagrada Família church trying to get a picture that captured it. Carolyn finally got a shot that captured the church in a totally fantasy way.

While she was looking for the perfect shot, I was taking a few also, but most of mine were of her, my favorite subject.

Research has shown that being creative helps make you happier, less anxious, more resilient and better equipped to problem-solve in the face of hardship, all good things when you are battling cancer.

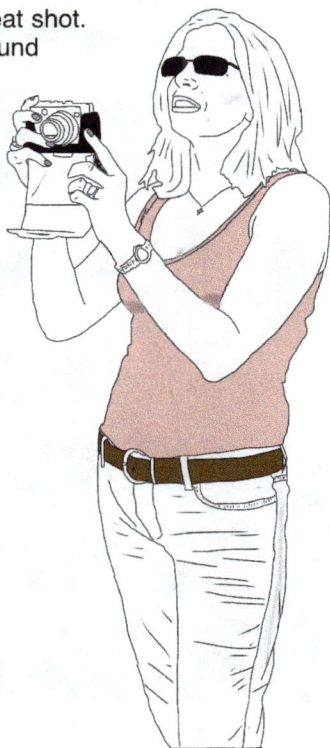

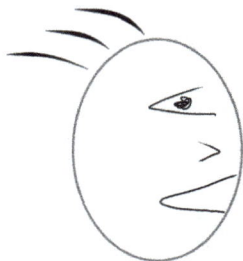

Taking pictures really forces you to focus on the moment.

Arrrgg, I'd really like to take a shot at, I mean shot of you right now!

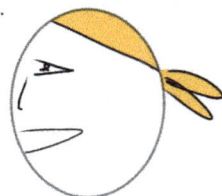

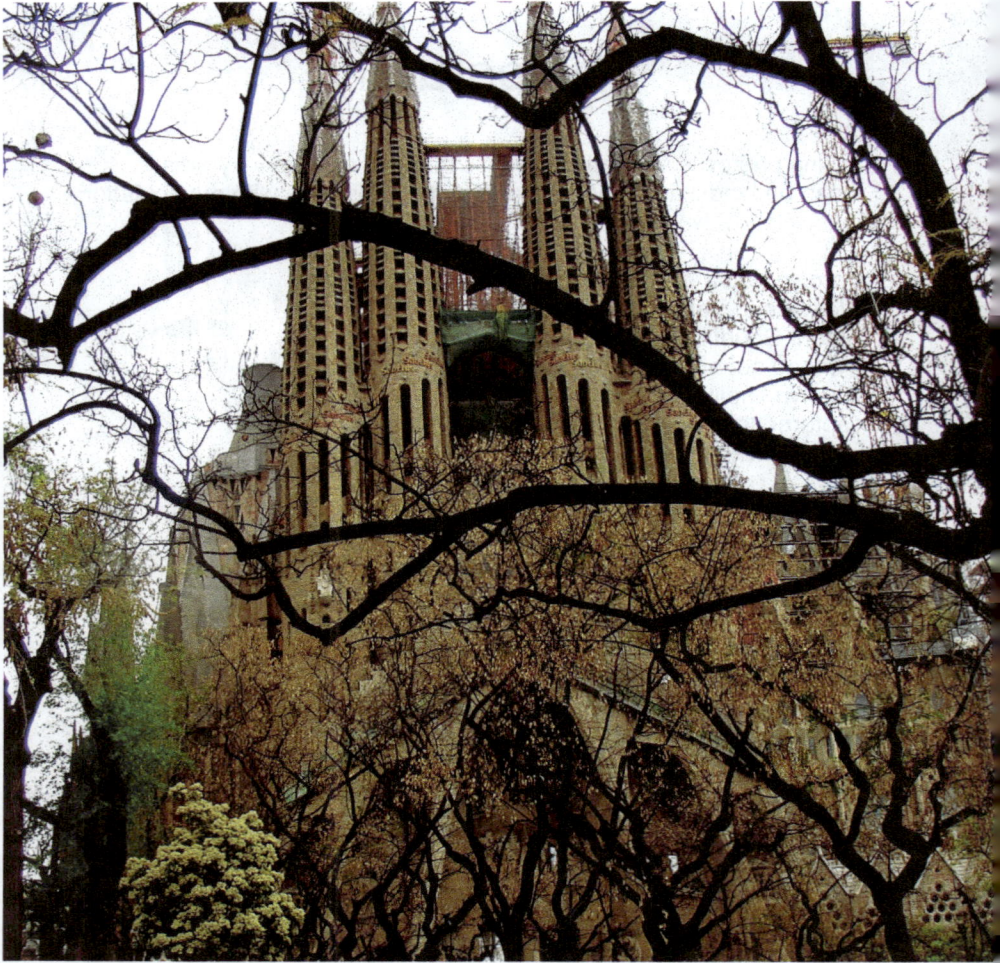

Cooking

We switched to all organic food when Carolyn was diagnosed with breast cancer. This included free range meat with no growth hormones or antibiotics whenever possible. We did not change to any type of extreme diet such as going vegan or juicing. Carolyn did truly love cooking and really good food is one of the pleasures of life.

Although she would deny it, she was a chef in my opinion. She would always heat the plates so the food wold be hot when it was served. She usually cooked from scratch and especially loved baking, such as...

o Perfecting the lemon-poppy scone.
o The "to die for" dark chocolate cake.
o Janes blueberry pie
o An exquisite tapas plate with drinks.
o Roasted Rosemary nuts (with rosemary that she grew).

Sweet is one of the last tastes to go when you are on chemo for an extended period of time, so desserts were satisfying. There is no scientific research that shows eating sugar "feeds" the cancer cells, or that cutting sugar from your diet will stop the cancer cells from dividing.

BUT, it is definitely worthwhile to eat as healthy as possible

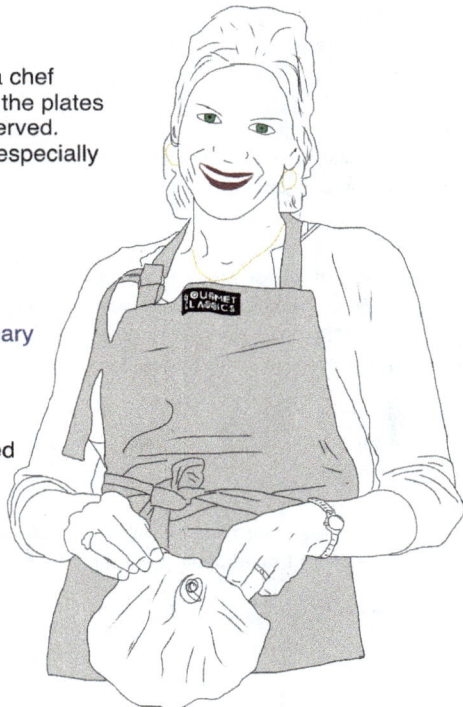

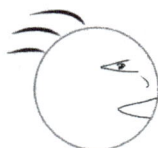

Eating to cure cancer is a fruitless undertaking.

Ha ha, fruit is good for you and cutting fruit from your diet since it has natural sugar makes no sense.

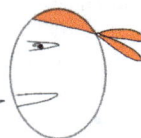

Recipes

The Perfect Lemon Poppy Scones

2 c. all-purpose flour
2 tbsp. sugar
2 tbsp. baking powder
1/2 tsp. soda
1/2 tsp. salt
1/4 c. butter, cut up
2/3 c. buttermilk
1 lg. egg
1 tbsp. poppy seeds
1 tsp. grated lemon peel

Combine dry ingredients in large mixing bowl. Cut in butter with pastry blender or 2 knives until mixture resembles coarse crumbs. Beat buttermilk and egg in small bowl. Pour onto dry ingredients. Add poppy seeds and lemon peel. Mix with fork until blended.

On lightly floured surface knead dough 5 or 6 times. Transfer to greased cookie sheet and pat into 8 inch circle with floured hands. Cut into 8 wedges with long sharp floured knife-do not separate. Bake 14-16 minutes in a 425 degree oven until golden brown.
Brush topping over top of hot scones. Serve warm.

TOPPING:
4 tbsp. sugar
2 tbsp. lemon juice

For Cheddar-Chive Scones: Reduce sugar to 1 tablespoon, omit poppy seed and lemon peel. Add Cheddar cheese (shredded), 1 tablespoon chives, omit topping.

Janes Blueberry Pie

1/2 cup water
1/2 cup sugar
1 quart blueberries (18 oz.)
2 tablespoons corn starch
2 tablespoons water
1 baked pie shell (Pillsbury is good)

In a pan heat 1/2 cup water & sugar until sugar dissolves, add 1 cup blueberries & bring to a boil.
Mix water & corn starch, add to blueberry mix.
Boil until mixture thickens.
Cool a bit, then fold in remaining berries.
Put in pie shell & chill for a few hours.

The Perfect Gin & Tonic

1 ½ ounces of Bombay Sapphire Gin
¼ lime
4 ounces Canadian Club tonic water

In a highball glass, fill with ice
Add the gin, then the lime and finally the tonic.
Garnish with a slice of lime on the rim and a swizzle stick.
Serve with a flourish on a tray with the glass sitting on a small napkin.

The "to die for" Deep Dark Chocolate Cake

1 3/4 cup flour	2 eggs
2 cups sugar	1 cup milk
3/4 cup coco	1/2 cup Veg. oil
1 1/2 tsp baking soda	2 tsp vanilla
1 1/2 bsp baking powder	1 cup boiling water
1 tsp salt	

Combine dry ingredients in a large mixing bowl.
Add remaining ingredients except boiling water.
Beat at medium speed for 2 minutes.
Stir in boiling water (batter will be thin).

Pour into two greased 9" pans or 1 13x9 pan.
Bake at 350 for 30-35 minutes.

FROSTING.
Beat 1 cup milk and a small box of instant chocolate pudding for 1 minute.
Fold in 1 8oz carton of Cool Whip and frost cake immediately and refrigerate!

The Perfect Rosemary Nuts

1 lb nuts (preferably pecans)
2 tbsp rosemary
1/2 tsp red or hot pepper
2 tsp dark brown sugar
2 tsp kosher salt / Big grained salt
1 tbsp 1/2 butter, 1/2 olive oil melted

Mix and pour over nuts
Spread on sheet
Bake at 350 degrees for 10 minutes

Chemotherapy Roulette

You never know what the side effects are going to be when you start a new chemo.
They may be tolerable or they may be intolerable.
Be it nausea, headaches, neuropathy, flu symptoms, or just mild discomfort.

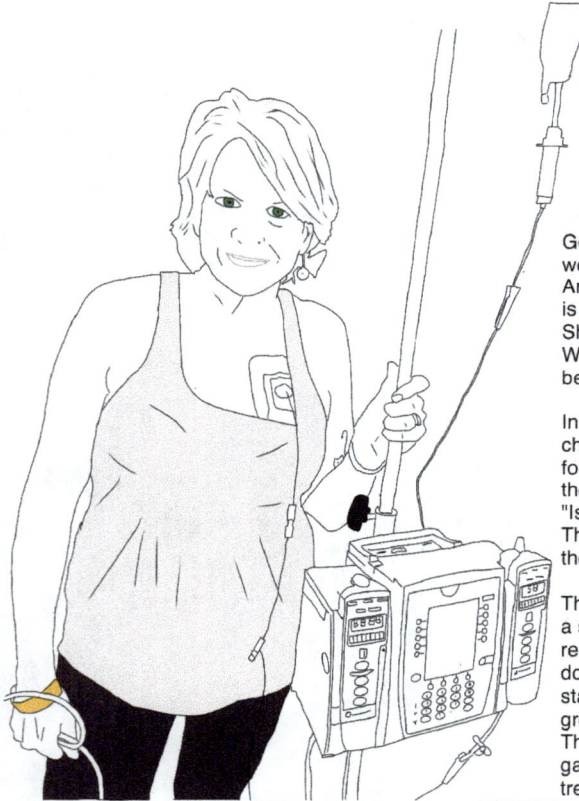

It is basically a spin of the wheel. Carolyn handled most of the treatments fairly well.
For instance Navelbine was easy on her until the neuropathy built up enough that she had to quit.

Genetic testing indicated that Afinitor would be a good treatment match for her. An uncommon side effect of this chemo is aggression and abnormal behavior. She got this side effect in spades! We quit the daily pills after two weeks because it was driving her crazy.

In fact, several weeks after we quit this chemo, Carolyn was put into twilight sleep for a broncoscopy. During the procedure, the surgeon turned to me and asked, "Is she always so agitated and combative?" The side effects had faded, but were still there.

The other way that each chemotherapy is a spin of the wheel is how well the cancer responds to the treatment. Some will knock down the tumors, some will just keep them stable, some will just slow down the tumor growth and some just won't help at all. That's why we had so many scans to gauge the effectiveness of the current treatment.

What if your standard treatment options are running out and you want to gamble on a long shot?

Well then you can try a drug trial. That is a good reason to get treatment at a research hospital. You won't know the effectiveness of the drug, and you won't know if your body will respond to it either.

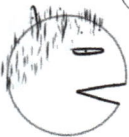

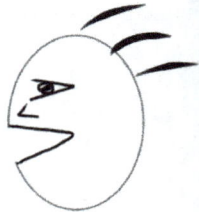

Working

Continuing to work while on chemotherapy depends on how well you feel after the infusions and how much you love your job. If you love your job, then continuing to work makes your life seem to be less turned upside down.

Although Carolyn was a trained Nurses Aide and a certified trainer, her primary job was a housewife. She enjoyed doing laundry, handling the warm clothes, folding and putting them away. She had the benefit of working from home so she did not have to get dressed up and go out to a job.

Her dressing up to go out was grocery shopping, where she would diligently compare prices, compare expiration dates, examine labels for healthy content and plan our meals. She got a lot of satisfaction in doing this and was good at it.

If you are working a job in an office or business, then it will be a bit more difficult, but not impossible. Although I did not have cancer and was not on chemotherapy, I went with Carolyn to most of her infusions, Dr visits, scans, procedures and surgeries. I did this by arranging to work from home and having flex hours. In fact I got some of my best work done in infusion while the drugs were dripping into her veins.

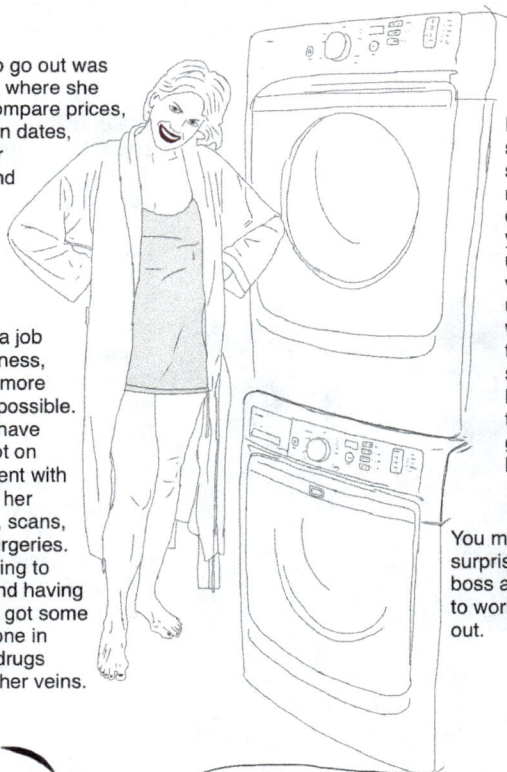

If you don't have strong support from your spouse, or your job has no flexibility in hours or work location, then you will be forced to use sick days and even vacation days to make up for the time off you will need during the treatment days. If your spouse is working and has good insurance, then now might be a good time to take a break from working.

You might be very pleasantly surprised at how much your boss and company are willing to work with you and help you out.

So, you really love your job as a housewife?

Yeah, and there's nothing like working in your robe!

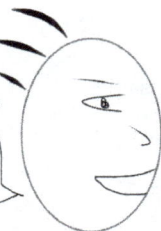

Well doing dishes, cleaning floors and bathrooms are not so much fun but the things I enjoy, like shopping for household goods makes up for it.

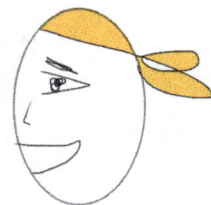

Wigs

If you are on chemo odds are that eventually you will be on one that will make you lose your hair. If you don't like hats or you don't like scarves, bandanas, buffs, or you don't like going around bald, then your best option is to get a wig.

Many wigs are made of synthetic hair, but these can look Halloween-like. The best wigs are made from human hair and these can look very natural. When going out no one would guess that it is not your actual hair. These are very pricey however and even wigs can be a bother on your head like a hat can be.

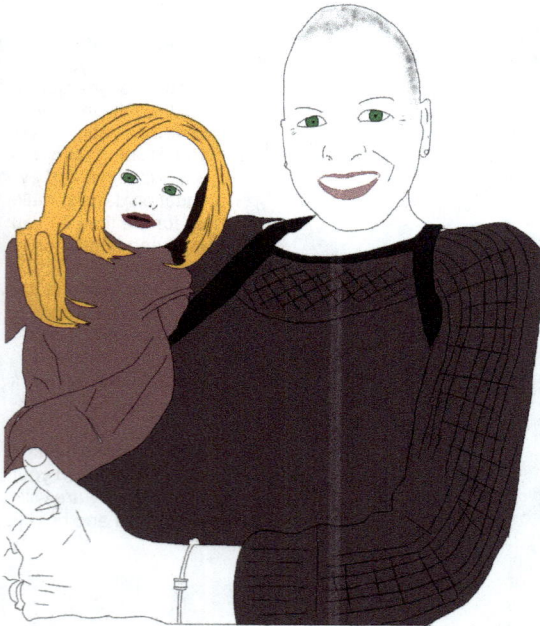

We ended up buying a wig from a wig shop. It was fun trying them on because it is amazing how much it can change your look.

Carolyn was very worried when she lost her hair that the grandkids would be scared of her. She eased into it with them by wearing her wig and making it plaything for her and the kids. This made it fun and non-threatening to them until eventually she quit wearing the wig altogether at home.

One cool thing is that you may be able to have your insurance company pay for part of the wig. We found it to be quite a hassle to get through all the approvals, referrals and paperwork of getting some reimbursement back.

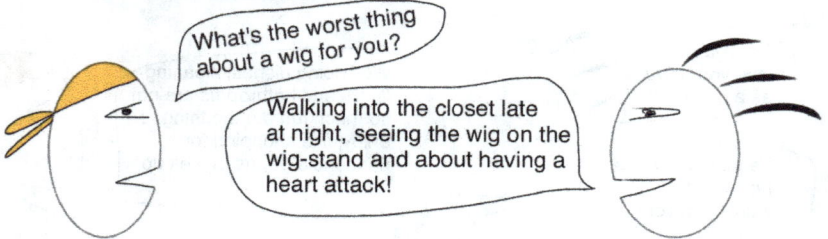

What's the worst thing about a wig for you?

Walking into the closet late at night, seeing the wig on the wig-stand and about having a heart attack!

Socializing

Recurring social events that you are a key part of, is a good way to keep up your contacts with friends and get you out of the house when you might be feeling lethargic.

Carolyn started the Stratford Lakes book club prior to her breast cancer diagnosis and continued with it until we eventually moved from the suburbs into the foothills. Not only would she enjoy the discussions and conversations at the meetings, but she would also discuss them with me since I would read them also. This was a woman's club with the exception being the occasional party with the husbands.

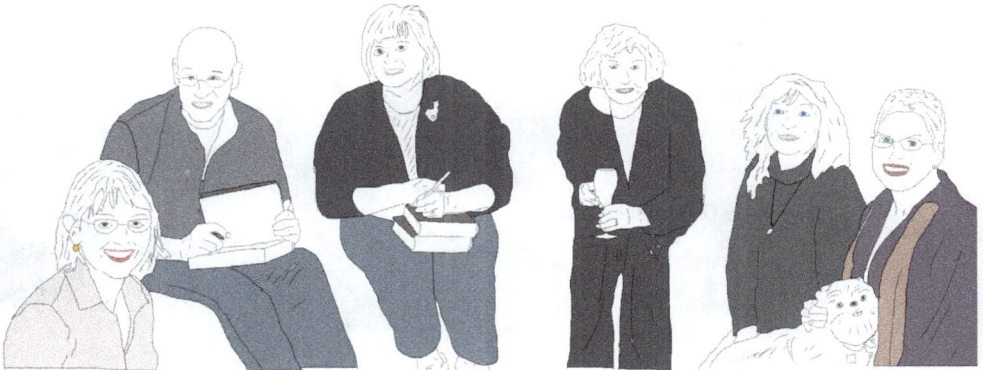

This particular meeting was discussing "The Story of Edgar Sawtelle" with the author David Wroblewski. At this meeting, Carolyn was on steriods to counteract the effects of a harsh chemo that she was on. She is still extremely beautiful, although you can see that her face is full and puffy from the steriod side-effects.

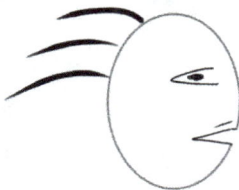

It is just a double whammy to have side-effects from your drug to alleviate the side-effects. At least the steriod side-effects mostly go away.

Music

Music cannot heal cancer, but it can sure make you feel better for the moment. It can be used to trigger nostalgic memories of good times in the past or reinforce a current feeling by really getting into the mood with songs that reinforce it.

Sometimes it's just an escape when it makes you get up and dance around enjoying it. We liked playing DJ for a minute where we would each choose a song that we liked, or one that we knew the other liked and would switch back and forth for hours having fun together.

Her favorite music ran the gambit including
Bee Gees
Van Morrison
South Park Mexican
The Beatles
Leonard Cohen
The Guess Who
Amy Winehouse
DC Talk
Weezer
Sarah McLachlan
Chicago
Creedence Clearwater Revival
Chris Isaak
The Cranberries
The Doors
George Harrison
House of Pain
It's a Beautiful Day
John Mayer
Michael Jackson
Harry Nilsson
Johnny Cash

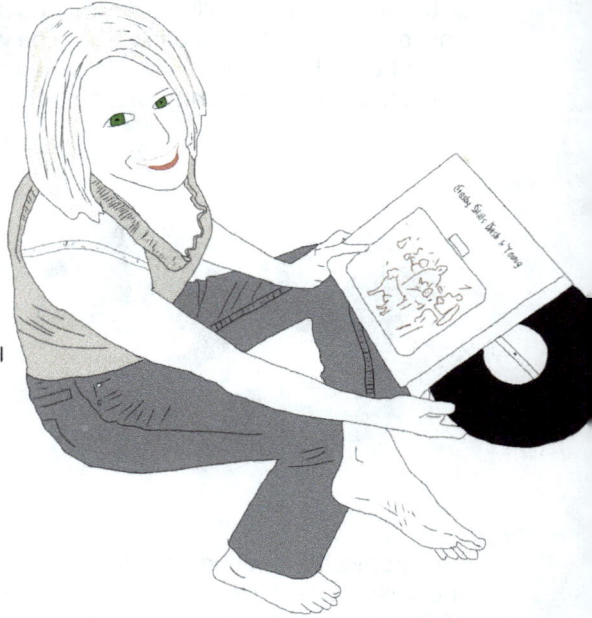

The song that I would consider "Our Song" is Wonderful, by Adam Ant.

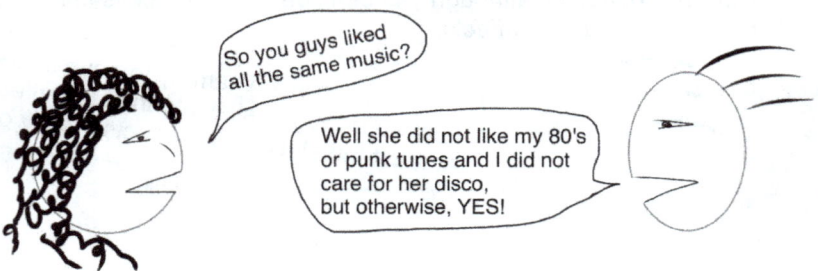

So you guys liked all the same music?

Well she did not like my 80's or punk tunes and I did not care for her disco, but otherwise, YES!

Having Fun

Carolyn thought it was odd that I would often end phone conversations with "Have fun". If you can have fun with what you are doing then why not! She seldom had trouble having fun, even in chemo treatments talking and joking with the nurses and surfing the net on her iPad.

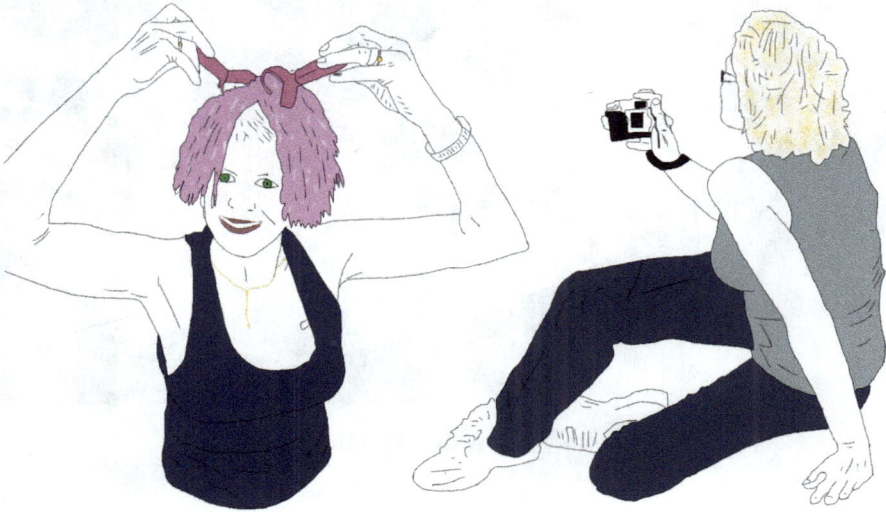

Of course you will always have down periods, since the disease and thoughts about death are always in the back of your mind. The fun times, even little bits of silliness can help keep depression at bay.

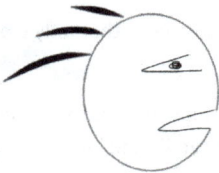

It might take a little Effexor or Wellbutrin however to help keep the fun alive!

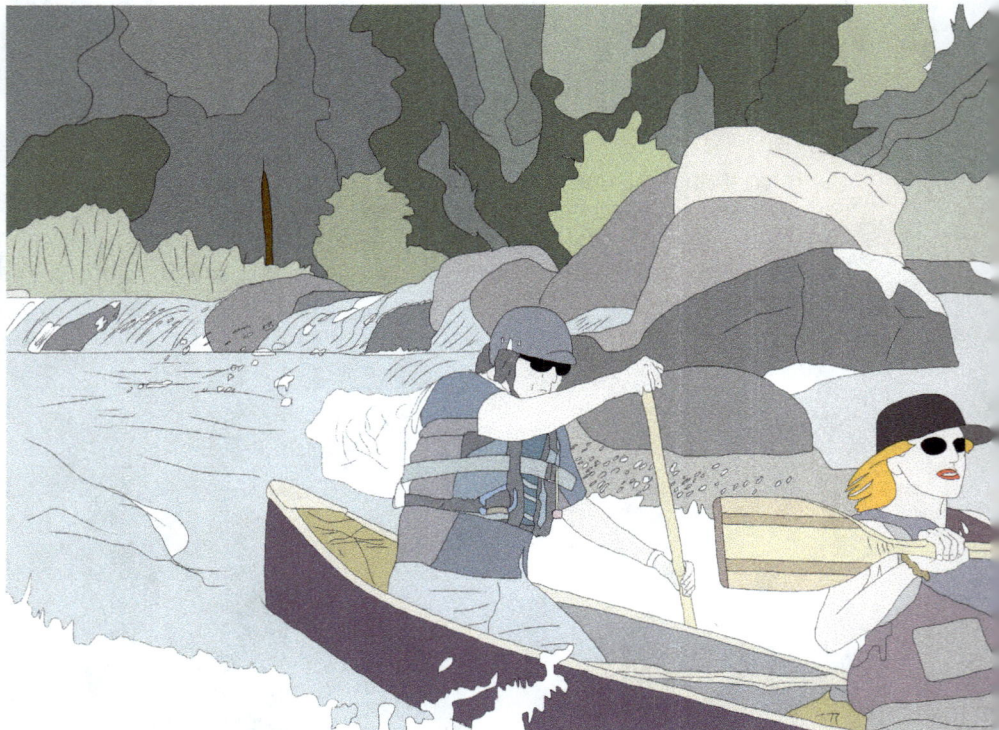

Tandem Whitewater Paddling

We started canoeing whitewater together before Carolyn was diagnosed with breast cancer. We would paddle on the lakes and work on the different paddling strokes and working together as a team to move the boat where we wanted to. We became proficient in forward and reverse strokes, draws, cross-bow draws, skulling, low and high braces, prys, j-strokes and quickly switching sides. These skills translated in our river paddling into eddy turns, peel-outs, surfing and safely running class 3 rapids together.

Paddling can really bring a couple together since it is like a ballet on the water that only works if both parties are relaxed and in harmony with each other.

If Carolyn was feeling good, we could paddle the local rivers such as the South Platte or the Colorado River and if she was not feeling on her "A" game, we could paddle the local lakes and have a relaxing time together. You can really pack a lot of items for a picnic into a canoe.

Something To Look Forward To

Anticipating something that you enjoy can help keep interest and joy in your life. Here we are celebrating the tickets we just bought for a trip to Paris and Barcelona. Besides going on the trip, she enjoyed all the planning leading up to the trip as well.

Carolyn would sometimes worry that we were spending too much money on trips to Europe, Vegas, Mexico, New York, etc., since she was a money manager at heart. I would put her at ease by telling her that any extra money spent on these excursions was coming from her part our retirement fund that she would never get to benefit from if we did not use it now.

You can see in this picture that Carolyn's hair had grown back nicely since she had been on several chemos that did not cause you to lose your hair. Her eyebrows came back so fine and light that they were hard to see.

You also have fun stuff after the trip, playing with your photos, giving gifts from the trip to the kids and grandkids and telling stories of your adventures.

But what if you don't like to travel?

Well there are plenty of other thing like getting a new camper and planning summer trips in it, getting a motorcycle and planning rides, remodeling a room exactly as you like it, or anything you like.

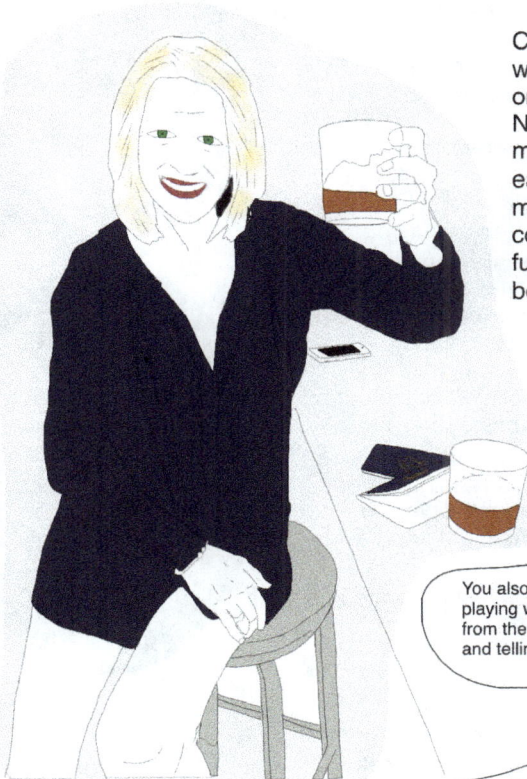

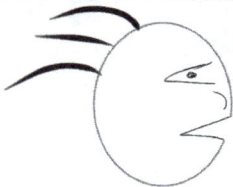

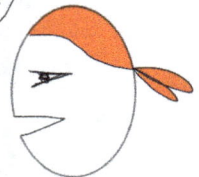

The Next Woman

I want to talk about the next woman after I'm gone.

Ummm, I'd rather not.

I've always been boy-crazy and I know that you have always been girl-crazy too. You may wait 3 days or 3 months but you won't wait years.

Let's talk about who your next woman should be.

No, there's only you.

Don't just go for a pretty face or a nice body, but find someone that you can really connect with and could possibly be another soulmate.

Ummm...

She should be a Christian woman about your age.

I'm not really comfortable with this.

She needs to be attractive and take care of herself. I think a former housewife would be perfect but not a career woman that does not really need a man.

Yeah, I suppose.

She should like to travel, like a little excitement and be capable of deep conversations, enjoy music, dancing and love to read.

Music and reading is good.

She should be smart, have her own opinions, love to snuggle and talk long into the night and be conservative.

Baby, you just described yourself

She needs to be feminine and dress nicely.
Someone whose advice you can trust...

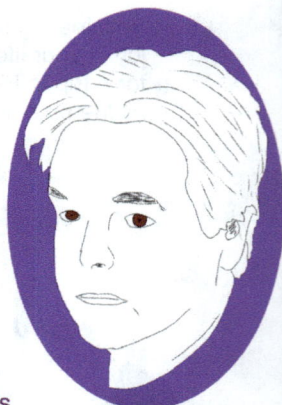

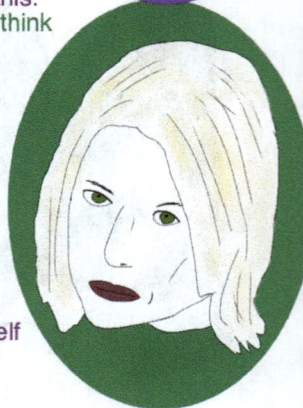

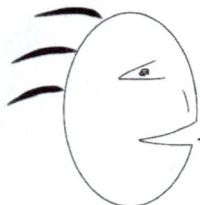

You do see that this conversation is just her way of trying to look after you and take care of you when she is gone.

Yeah, I suppose you are right.
Anyone that knows her, knows the futility of not discussing something she has on her mind.

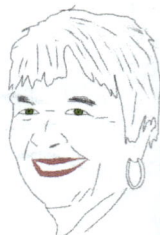

Fun in the Sun

Chemotherapy and especially radiation treatment will make your skin more sensitive to the sun and you will burn easier. The chemo will also dry out your skin so you don't have all the natural skin oils making the sun a double whammy.

That means wearing hats outside, wearing lots of sunscreen and beach coverups. An umbrella on the beach is probably the best thing you can do.

Don't be scared to be out in the sun for brief periods but don't be surprised if you get some cute freckles that you never had before.

Always wear dark sunglasses when out in the bright sunshine since many chemo drugs will make your eyes more sensitive to the light and some will cause your eye lashes to fall out or get thinner, reducing your natural eye protection from the sun.

Here Carolyn is wearing a big floppy hat to protect her face, neck and shoulders from the sun and drinking LOTS of fluids to stay hydrated

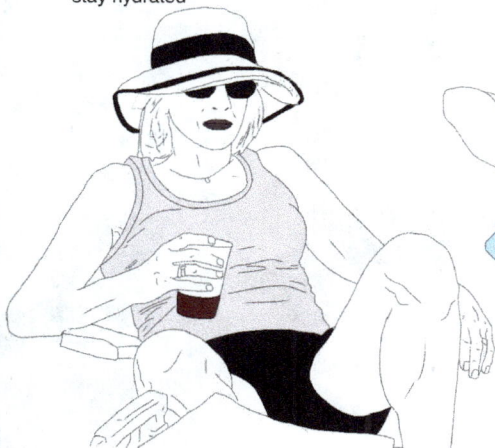

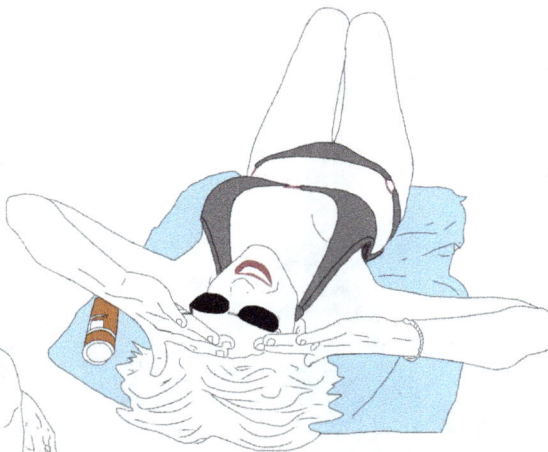

After a dip in the chilly North Atlantic off of Cape Cod, Carolyn is warming up on a towel, but is also liberally applying sunscreen.

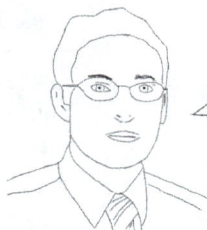

So Doc, is it best to just apply liberal amounts of sunscreen whenever I'm out in the sun.

The best thing to do is just stay out of the sun entirely.

Ok, so liberal amounts of sunscreen it is!

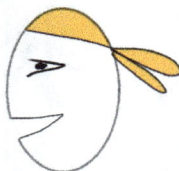

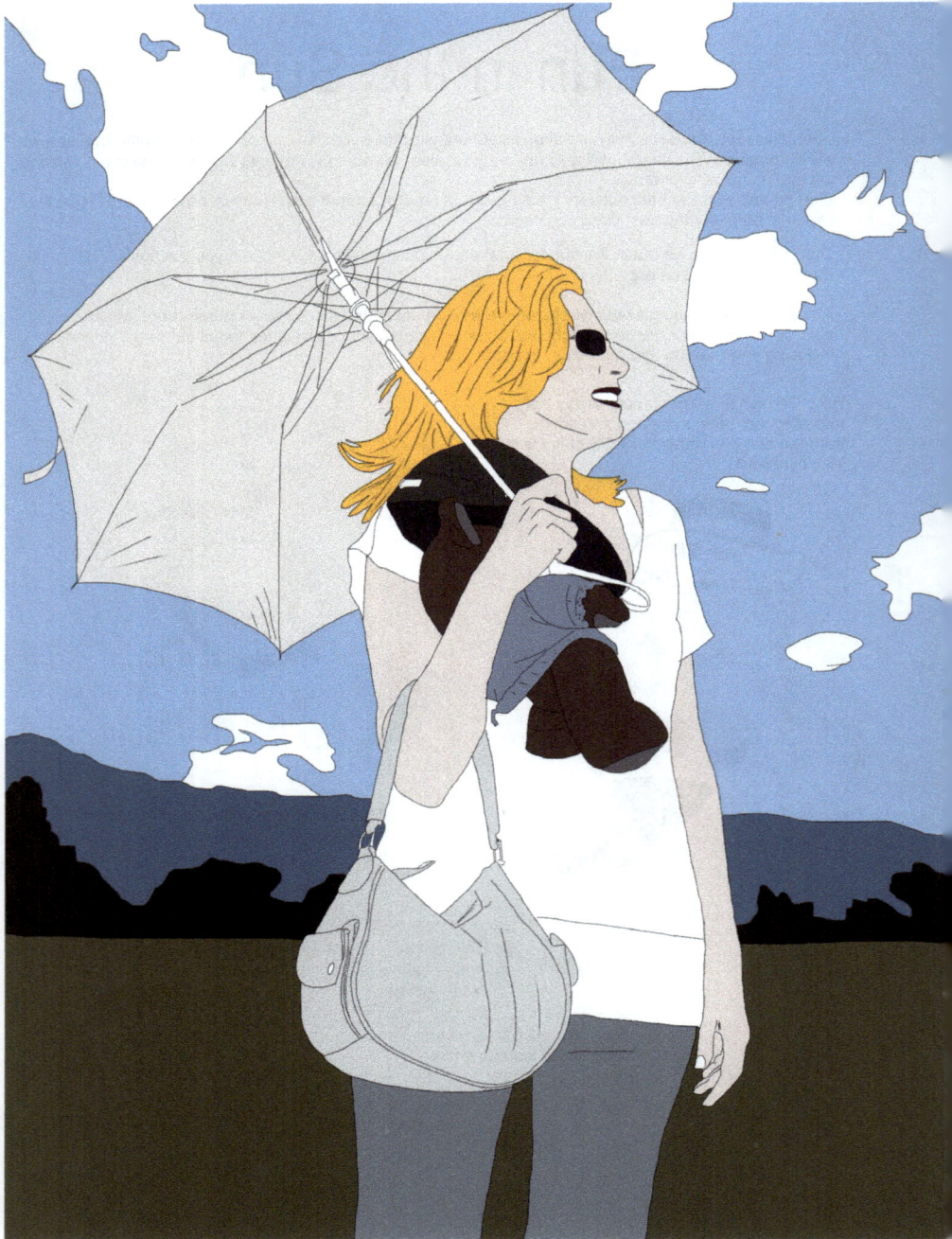

Mothers and Daughters

Having a close friend that you can confide in and discuss whatever is on your mind is a wonderful part of your support network. Carolyn had a number of very close friends. Her closest friend was her daughter Hailey. They would talk and text on and off every day, occasionally to the annoyance of others.

A daughter can closely relate to topics such as kids and her grandkids, husbands, siblings, financial issues, politics, television, vacations, school and so forth. Really any topic could be up for discussion in a depth that only a daughter can truly understand.

Not only would they support each other, but Carolyn would give Hailey advice on raising her kids and supporting her young family. Carolyn would spend time thinking about (and talking with me about) how she could help and advise Hailey. This would take her mind off the cancer, chemo treatments and thoughts of her uncertain future. It's funny how having something else to worry about can be such a good thing.

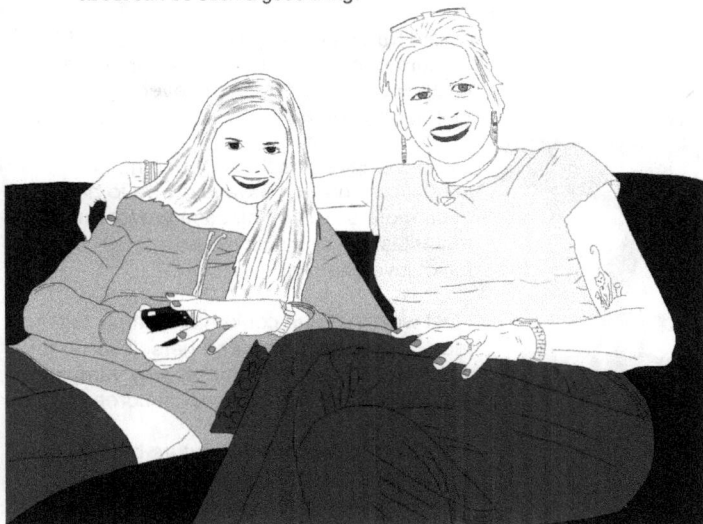

Carolyn talked to Hailey and I often about what she wanted for herself in case of a medical emergency and end of life care. Carolyn trusted us completely to carry out her wishes so we both carried little medical Power Of Attorney forms for Carolyn. We took,the big legal form and scaled it down to a tiny (but still legal) size that would fit in our wallets.

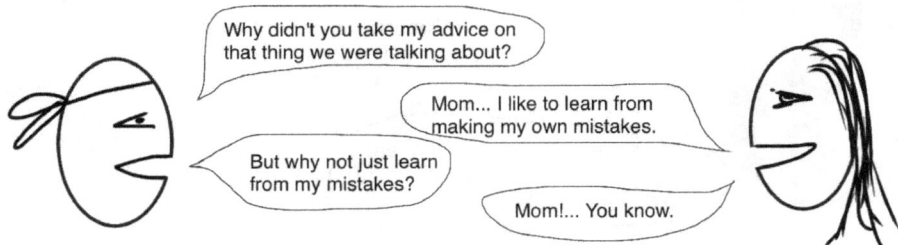

Why didn't you take my advice on that thing we were talking about?

Mom... I like to learn from making my own mistakes.

But why not just learn from my mistakes?

Mom!... You know.

Chemo Vampires

When we are home, Carolyn liked to be in a dark place. Not mentally, but physically. The chemo does make you sensitive to light and especially after being out during the day, you just crave a reprieve from the sun. The upstairs of our house is extremely open, bright and sunny. As the chemo treatments wore on, her favorite room of the house migrated to our downstairs family room which only has one small window that can be shuddered.

If the lamps are not on dimmers, then a light scarf can be draped over them, providing a gentle relaxing filtered light. It might just be a coincidence, but Carolyn did not care for garlic, saying that it gave us bad breath but for some pasta dishes we just had to.

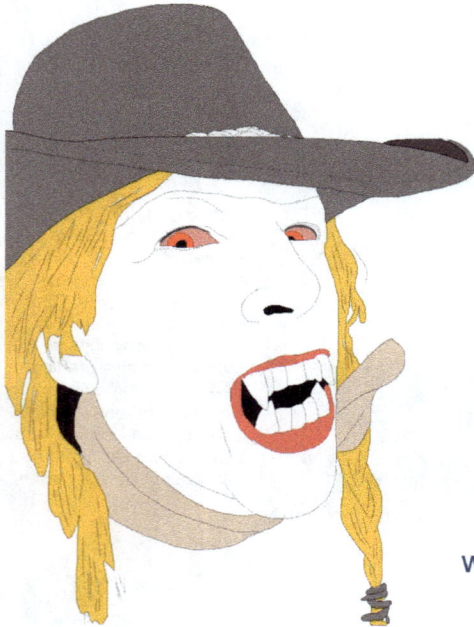

Unlike true vampires, we slowly tapered off our nighttime outings since her energy levels would be lower in the evening than during the day.

Like a vampire however, I found her irresistible and was always drawn to her, even more so as the disease progressed, metastasized and showed how tough and full of love she really was.

I just wish that she could have simply bitten me on the neck, and cured herself, living for another 100 years, but that is why vampires are just fantasy. Oh well, we can dream.

The reality is science and future break-throughs leading to a cure. Even now, Carolyn is helping future women with her research grant at

www.cufund.org/CarolynBidwell

Donate and leave a comment if you are so inclined!

It is actually the nurses that are much more likely to say, "I vaunt to dwraw your blood".

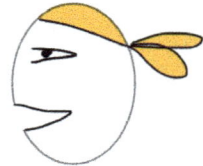

Contrary Carrie

When Carolyn was a little girl, she would get in these moods where she would not do what her parents wanted. At those times, they would call her "Contrary Carrie". Dealing with cancer, chemotherapy, surgeries and life issues wears on you eventually and occasionally Contrary Carrie would reemerge.

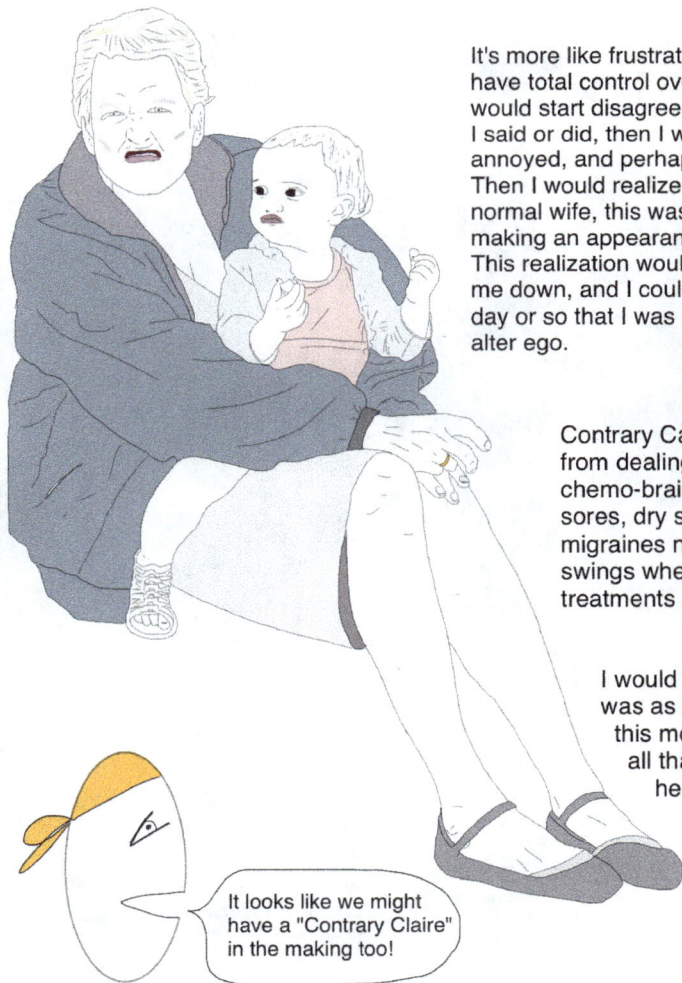

It's more like frustration that you no longer have total control over your life. When she would start disagreeing with everything that I said or did, then I would start getting annoyed, and perhaps a little pissed off. Then I would realize that this is not my normal wife, this was Contrary Carrie making an appearance to help her cope. This realization would immediately calm me down, and I could deal with it for the day or so that I was hanging out with her alter ego.

Contrary Carrie was a relief valve from dealing with things like chemo-brain, occasional mouth sores, dry skin, neuropathy and migraines not to mention mood swings when certain chemo treatments required steroids.

I would think how cute she was as a little girl being in this mood and I would see all that same cuteness in her as a grown woman.

It looks like we might have a "Contrary Claire" in the making too!

Dog Walks

One of the benefits of dog ownership is that they need to be taken on a walk every day. The dog will bug you everyday to take him on a walk. It is like having a workout partner that bugs you not to skip a day. Besides getting you out of the house and getting some exercise yourself, you can see the pleasure on your dogs face.

If you are going on a walk, the dog probably needs to be on a leash, but on a hike you can let him run free and can walk unencumbered. We are extremely fortunate to live in an area where we can take interesting walks and hikes right from our back door. Here Carolyn is hiking a couple of ridges away from our house. Dillon just cannot take his eyes off of the view of the Centennial Cone.

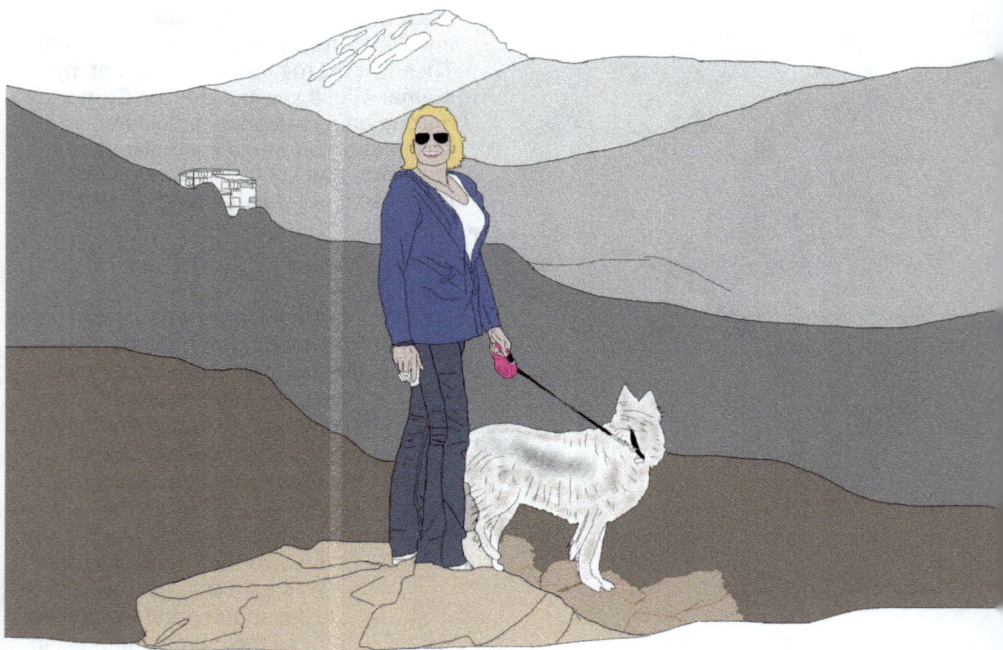

Studies have shown that pet owners exhibit decreased blood pressure, cholesterol and triglyceride levels. This can only be a benefit especially when you are undergoing a chemo treatment like the wonder-drug Herceptin that can eradicate your Her-2 positive breast cancer, but will also cause heart damage in the process.

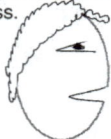

But what if I'm allergic to dogs or there are no pets allowed at my place or I'm just not a dog person?

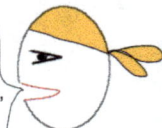

Well you will just have to motivate yourself to take those daily walks. Perhaps a friend, spouse, child, or heaven forbid, by yourself. Good luck taking a cat on a walk.

Gossip - Word of Mouth

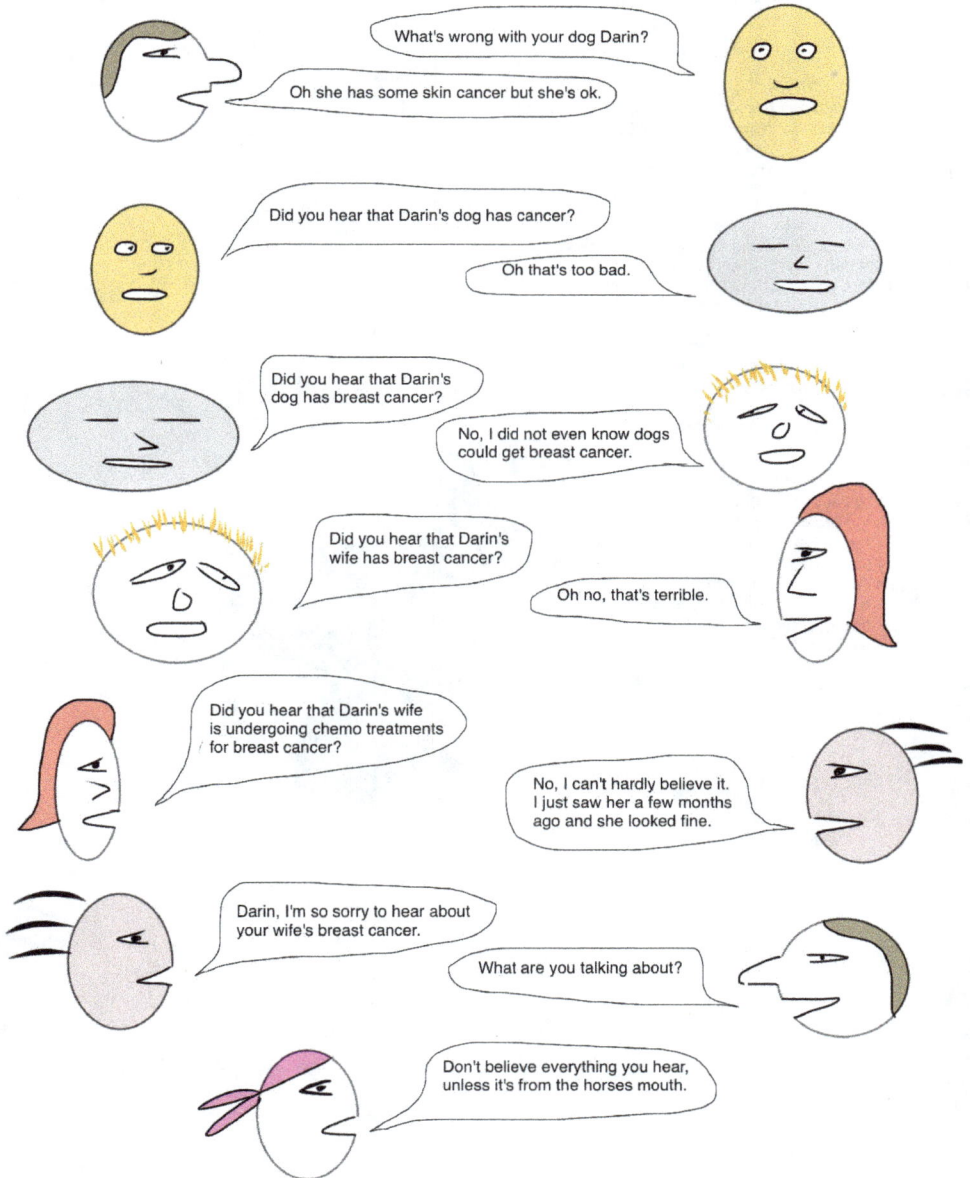

What's wrong with your dog Darin?

Oh she has some skin cancer but she's ok.

Did you hear that Darin's dog has cancer?

Oh that's too bad.

Did you hear that Darin's dog has breast cancer?

No, I did not even know dogs could get breast cancer.

Did you hear that Darin's wife has breast cancer?

Oh no, that's terrible.

Did you hear that Darin's wife is undergoing chemo treatments for breast cancer?

No, I can't hardly believe it. I just saw her a few months ago and she looked fine.

Darin, I'm so sorry to hear about your wife's breast cancer.

What are you talking about?

Don't believe everything you hear, unless it's from the horses mouth.

Embrace Your Inner Child

Sometimes the most relaxing and satisfying thing you can do is something childish and creative. Rediscover some of the wonder of your childhood. Who cares what anyone thinks. You are a free spirit and this is just one way of expressing it.

Although you are totally a mature woman, what a compliment to be told that you are are girlish. Not just a cute girlish figure, but the fun carefree air of a playful girl that brings joy to all around you. What better way than to keep in touch with those things that you loved as a kid. Lord knows that you have enough grownup stuff to worry about.

Carolyn would always tell me stories about her as a girl growing up. She never forgot her childhood memories. For me it was like a window into the mysterious world of of girls that has always been a wonder to me.

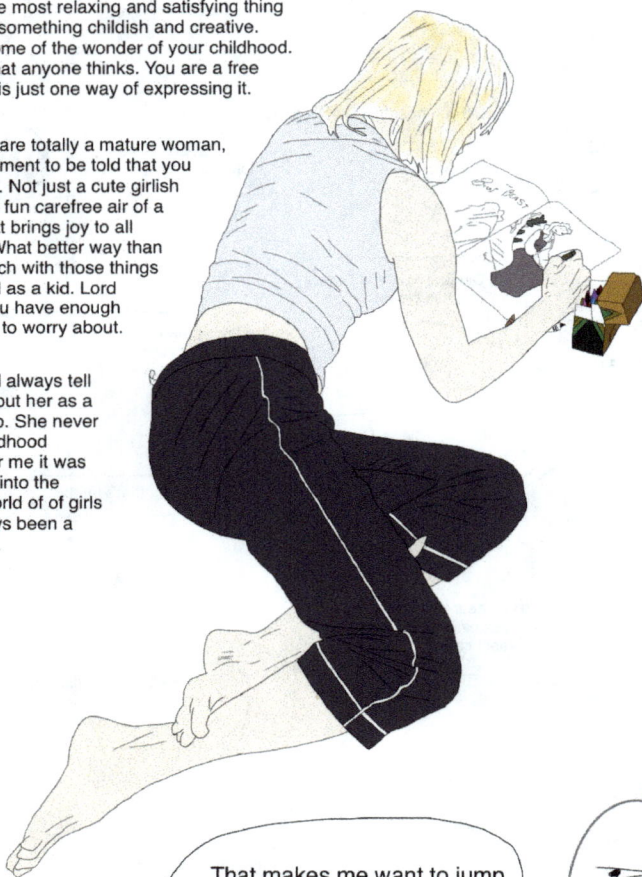

That makes me want to jump down onto the floor and do some coloring myself.

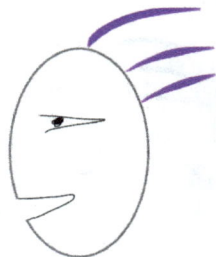

People Helping People

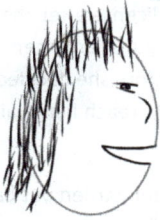

Hey Neighbor, how's your wife doing?

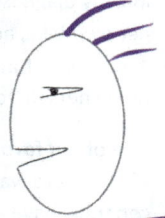

She's doing well considering, thanks for asking.

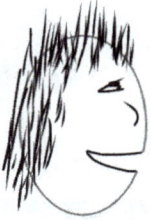

I'd like to help out by making you dinner tomorrow.

Well thank you. I'm not much of a cook, but my speciality is Mac & cheese. Plain, with extra cheese and peanuts, with steamed broccoli, and other variations. Carolyn is teaching me other dishes, but that is my go-to meal.

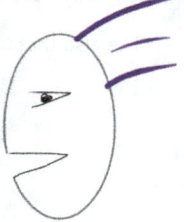

The next day...

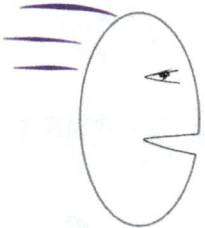

Hey Baby, I've got some dinner from out neighbor.

Excellent, it will be nice to have a real home cooked meal. What is it?

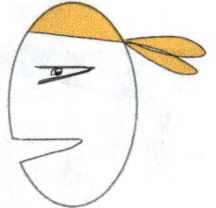

Mac & cheese...

Arrrg

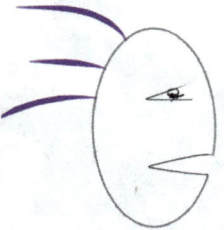

Hey, at least it's a variation I've never made with tuna and mushrooms.

Well, it IS Mac & cheese, but let's hope it's really Good Mac & cheese.

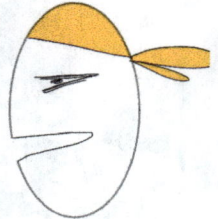

I should have told her that my speciality is Lobster Thermidor.

This print is one that I created for the Cancer Ride to raise money for Carolyn's Fund at the CU Cancer Center.

This has special meaning to me since Carolyn decided to get her Motorcycle license after she was initially diagnosed. She took a training class and successfully passed the riding test and then had her own bike, an 1100 Yamaha Virago. We rode for about a year together before she decided that it was more fun and comfortable to ride with me on the larger Harley. She did reach her goal of riding herself however.

One of our favorite destinations was The Buffalo Rose bar that has a biker beer garden out back where there was usually a band playing. We would listen to music, dance, talk to other bikers and generally have a good time there.

I like also that the avatars of Carolyn and I are talking in an upstairs room.

"Four wheels move your body, two wheels move your soul" - Carolyn

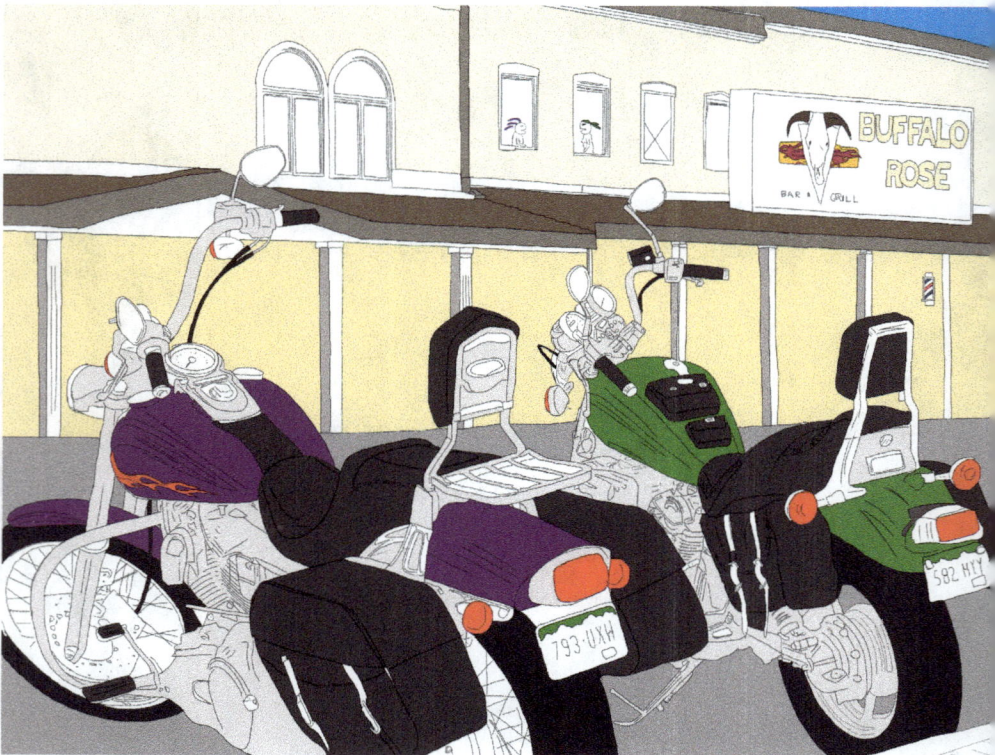

His and Hers

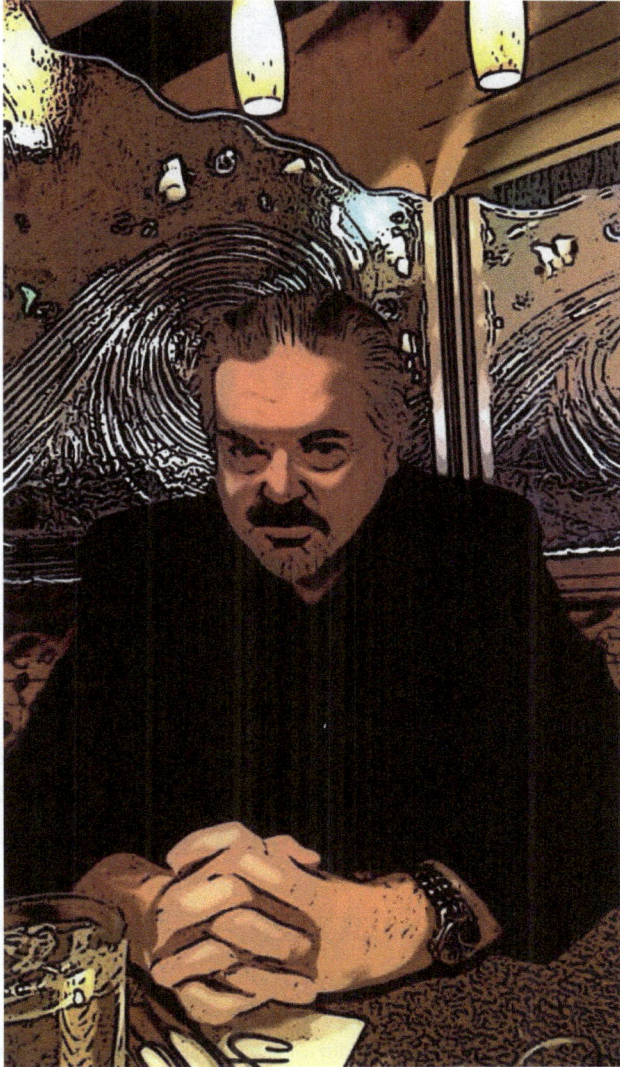

Carolyn took this tooncamera shot while we were out celebrating her latest scans. 2 of 3 brain tumors gone (the 3rd is 2/3s smaller), and the lung mets have shrunk. - December 12, 2013

CSB - And I'm a damn good photographer babe!

CFB - I don't often go out for a drink, but when I do I make sure it's happy hour.

Post Cancer Insights

Carolyn Bidwell Metastatic Breast Cancer Research Memorial Fund

The purpose of this memorial fund is to provide support to metastatic breast cancer research at the CU Canter Center at the discretion of Dr. Peter Kabos at the University of Colorado Anschutz Medical Campus in memory of Carolyn Bidwell.

Online Donations
The URL is www.cufund.org/CarolynBidwell

Donations by Check
If you would like to make a donation and would prefer to write a check, write them to: CU Foundation, and in the memo line write: Carolyn Bidwell Memorial Fund #0223914
Please mail the checks to:

Angela DellaSalle
13001 E. 17th Pl., MS AO65
Aurora, CO 80045

University of Colorado
Cancer Center
A NATIONAL CANCER INSTITUTE-DESIGNATED
CONSORTIUM COMPREHENSIVE CANCER CENTER

Carolyn Bidwell Memorial Ride for Cancer Research
I'm including a couple of the flyers that I did for the ride and celebration of Carolyn's life since there are images of her that Capture her spirit.

This will also be an annual event, and anyone can attend and/or do the ride.

First Annual Carolyn Bidwell Memorial Ride
for Cancer Research
Saturday, June 13 at 10:00 AM

If you have cancer, know anyone that has cancer, have lost someone to cancer or just want to support people fighting cancer, then this ride is for you. RSVP to ChristopherBidwell@gmail.com or just show up.

A $20 donation includes a wrist band for food specials and entry into a drawing for a piece of original artwork inspired by Carolyn. The 1st 100 riders also get a custom embroidered patch!

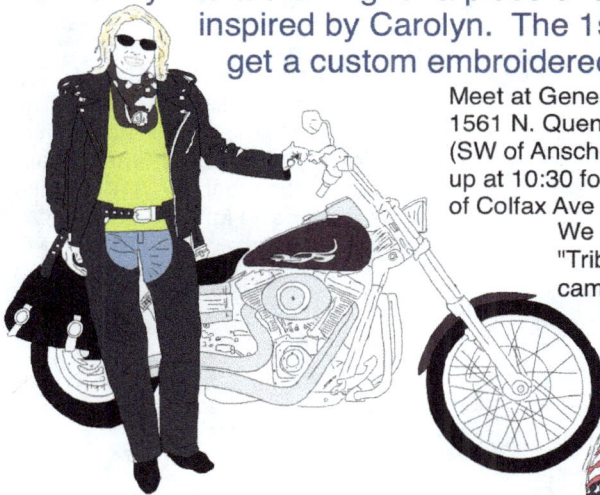

Meet at Generals Park at 1561 N. Quentin St, Aurora CO (SW of Anschutz on Colfax). Kickstands up at 10:30 for a ride down the length of Colfax Ave & into the foothills. We will end up at the the "Tributary at 244" for relaxation, camaraderie and fun on the deck to live music by the Platte River Band.

If you don't ride but you want to show your support, just show up at the Trib at 1:00 the afternoon

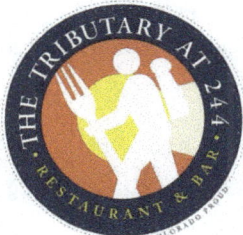

Proceeds from the event go to the Carolyn Bidwell Metastatic Breast Cancer Research Memorial Fund at the CU Cancer Center.

http://www.cufund.org/CarolynBidwell

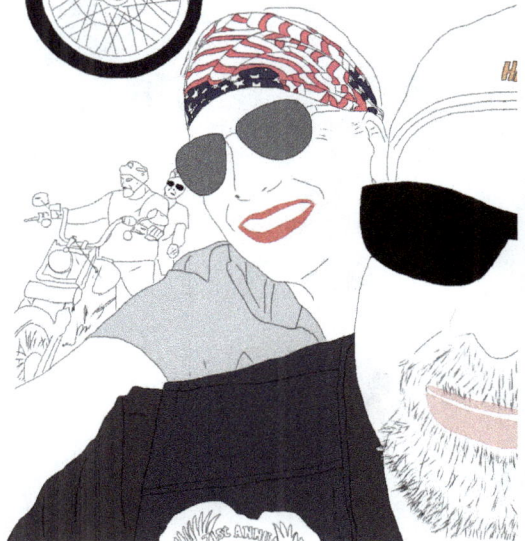

Carolyn Bidwell Celebration & Fund-Raiser

We are having a party to celebrate Carolyn and to raise money for her charity.

Saturday, June 13th at 1:00 PM at the Trib

Your $20 donation (at the Tributary at 244) will go directly to the
CAROLYN BIDWELL METASTATIC BREAST CANCER RESEARCH MEMORIAL FUND
www.cufund.org/CarolynBidwell and you get a wrist band for food specials
and will be entered into a drawing for a piece
of original artwork inspired by Carolyn.
There will also be rocking-good music from
the Platte River Band.

After-party, June 13 @ 7:00 PM

The after-party will also be at the Tributary
but will be more adult oriented with
the edgy Irish songs from the Pheasant
Pluckers, a local band. A $10 donation
gets a wrist band for food specials.
Any donations are welcome.

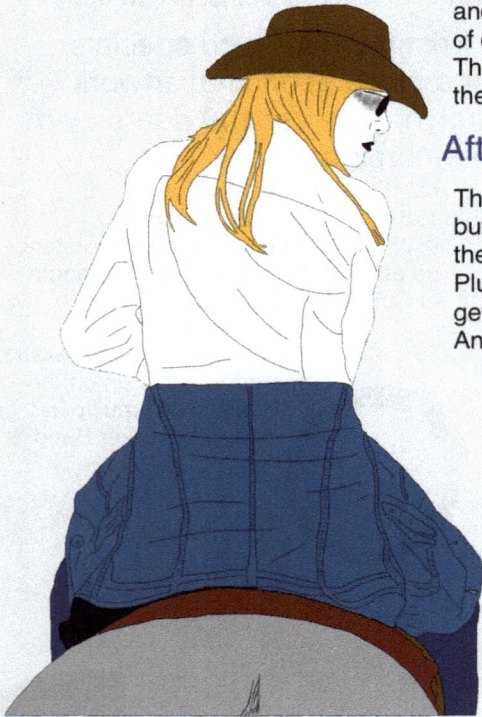

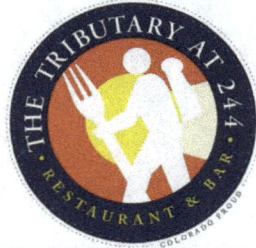

The Tributary at 244 Resturant
33295 US-6, Idaho Springs, CO
(Only 28 miles from Denver)

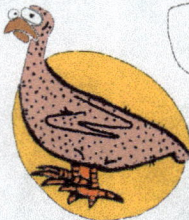

Forget your motorcycle,
I've got a horse outside!

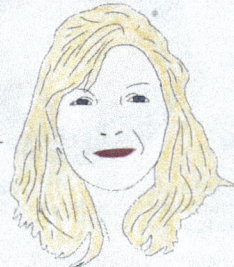

Acknowledgments

- www.cancer.gov
- www.breastcancer.org
- www.mayoclinic.org
- www.uch.uchealth.org/Breast-Cancer
- www.cancerresearchuk.org
- www.webmd.com/**breast-cancer**
- www.**epocrates**.com
- www.health.harvard.edu
- www.facebook.com
- ArtStudio IOS App

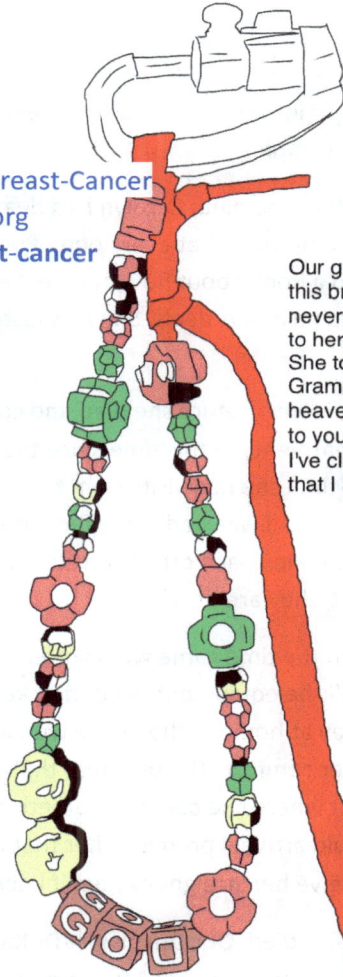

Our granddaughter Stella made this bracelet for Carolyn but never got a chance to give it to her before she died.
She told me "I made this for Gramma Bidwell but she is in heaven now. I want to give it to you".
I've clipped it on my man-bag that I always carry with me.

I would like to thank Dr. Peter Kabos for editing the initial manuscript.

I am grateful to Cynthia Girand for proofing the final manuscript.

I would like to thank Hailey Bussey for reviewing each page to ensure accuracy and as my touchstone for inclusion in the book.

Carolyn Bidwell reviewed many of these pages as they were being created.

Postscript

I feel that some thought into the end of life process is needed to make this account of our cancer journey complete.

In the last months before she died, Carolyn had death always in the back of her mind. It's weird that something that every one of us will go through is so wrapped in mystery. She had read a book about how people die from various diseases and most of them were long and painful ordeals. She was just hungry for knowledge so that she could plan.

She lost her voice the month before she died and could only whisper. We also quit the chemotherapy treatments at this time since the side effects just made breathing more difficult. At this time she had visits from her family and friends and got closure and goodbyes from them all. We had some fun with it as we would be whispering together like we were telling each other secrets. Someone would walk into the room and I would say "quiet, they are here".

We decided that when the time came we wanted to go to a real hospice facility with doctors, nurses and all the equipment needed to keep her the most comfortable. We also wanted her to stay at home in the house with all her pets that she loved and things that brought her comfort. The only fear that we both shared was that she would get to the point where she could not breath and would choke to death at home before help could arrive. I promised her that I would not let that happen on my watch and would give her straight oxygen if I needed to until help arrived.

Two days before Carolyn died, Our Oncologist Dr Kabos called and we upped the Dilaudid from every 12 hours to every 4 hours and doubled her steroid, both to help with her breathing difficulties. Carolyn cried on the phone when she told Dr Kabos that she loved him. She knew the end was near and Dr Kabos confirmed this by telling her she had perhaps a week left. He was being generous.

The next day we checked into the Lutheran Hospice that we had looked at earlier and had liked. When my mom and I were taking Carolyn into the hospice, she remarked as we were driving down our road that it was so good to get out. It was a beautiful clear fall day in the mountains and fall is Carolyn's favorite season. Carolyn had been mostly eating my cooking for the last few weeks and wanted to go to a drive- thru on the way. Her favorite fast food is a filet of fish sandwich at McDonalds so that's where we went since we could eat without getting out of the car.

Carolyn immediately felt relief in the hospice. We met with two doctors in the first few hours that we were there. The room was beautiful and there were nurses always just down the hall.

The next day Carolyn passed away very peacefully at 10:20 PM, asleep and on a low-level morphine drip. She never woke up from her first night sleeping in the hospice. Hailey and I sat with her all day. She was sleeping and we were just holding her hand, wiping her brow and adjusting her oxygen mask. Hailey had gone home a few hours earlier and I got up from her bedside to turn out the lights and was getting into the bed next to hers to go to sleep. The second that my head hit the pillow I knew that my wife was gone. I think that she was holding on while I was there talking with her and praying with her and comforting her. When I went to bed, that was her signal that she could let go and go to heaven. I got right back up and prayed over her and cried my first grief, but had a sense of relief also that she had died so peacefully and without the fear and pain that she had dreaded.

I take no credit for having Carolyn at home until the last possible moment in relative comfort and then having her in the hospice for less than two days before she died. It was the perfect scenario for us. God was surely watching over us. Thank you Lord.

Afterword

My two favorite times of day were both related to Carolyn.

The first is looking forward to morning, when we have our morning coffee together, talk about our dreams and plans for the day, relax and check up on the days events on our iPads and just enjoy being with each other.

The second is looking forward to going to bed and snuggling up to sleep. Carolyn loves to snuggle tight and so do I.

I had not really cried for anything since I was a boy of 12. I wondered how I would deal with Carolyn's death. It turns out that crying is not a problem. I would cry when hugging friends and family, even neighbors. I would cry when Dillon would run out to the car to greet Carolyn and be confused since she was not there, it was just me. I would cry when driving to work and singing songs that we liked together. I still have yet to get through a church service without crying, partly because the songs we sing bring me close to her and God and partly because that is where we held her service. Several friends had told me that things that you cannot foresee, even months or years later, would trigger the grieving. Some random thought will come into my mind, trigger an intense feeling about Carolyn and I will tear up and then talk and pray to her. They were right.

I had lots of friends and family staying with me for a few weeks after her death. A day or two after Carolyn died, late at night, shooting pool with my daughter Corinne, I stopped with the sudden realization that I needed to call Carolyn, thinking that she must be out of town visiting her sister or Hailey, then realizing...

Now that she is gone, I just want to hug her and sob in her arms. I did not really cry until she was gone however, just tearing up a couple of times when we talked about it.

Hugging and Crying

Carolyn and I talked about her eventual death from cancer and cried about it but mostly talked about it pragmatically.
After her death I sobbed, often weeks later when hugging family, friends and neighbors.

What I really wish were that I could sob my eyes out while hugging Carolyn and holding her tight. Just get it all out, crying together. She is the only one I really wanted to hug after her death.

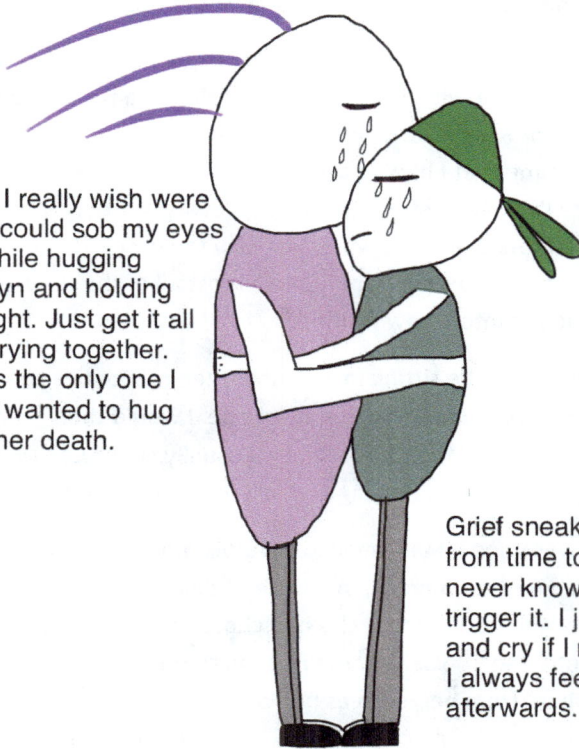

Grief sneaks up on you from time to time and you never know what will trigger it. I just go with it and cry if I need to. I always feel better afterwards.

My only concession to manhood and crying is to never accept a Kleenex when it is offered. Tissues are for girls I would tell myself. I just like to let my tears dry naturally on my cheeks like saline strips of remembrance for my baby.

The two main things that I do to deal with the grief are the spiritual counseling that I do. I have never been to any type of counseling and it is surprisingly enjoyable to just spend an hour or two talking about yourself. My counselor is also my pastor but he feels more like a friend that I could just have a beer with. He has given me so many insights into my life, my old life and my future life. The other thing that is a comfort is writing this book and working on the drawings about our life together.

Sleeping has been a problem since I cannot fall asleep without Carolyn next to me, even if I'm just touching her with a toe, it is comforting and relaxing and I can go right out. I only got 5 or 6 hours of sleep a night for the first month after she was gone. In fact the 1st time that I had a normal sleep was when I overslept (I had quit using an alarm since I've been getting up at 5 or 6 every morning after going to bed after midnight) on a Monday when I was going into the office. I had started going into work most days after working from home almost all of the time. It is good to get out of the house and get into a new routine.

Sometimes at work I would be sitting in my cube, then realize I've spent the last 20 minutes just looking at pictures of her on my phone. I would then go into an empty office to be alone and realize that this is where I usually called Carolyn from several times a day. Finally I would pack my bag and just leave work in the middle of the day.

A month after she was gone I finally mailed a Netflix movie that had been sitting on the dresser and I had never watched.   A couple of days later, I got a surprise movie in the mail what was the last one that she had chosen and put into our queue. The movie was Gods Not Dead. It was very meaningful to me as I watched it. I continue to get little "messages" from her, such as her last email that she never sent, a Pinterest message to me with a note and picture about a romantic evening we had on a London rooftop and a last list for Costco that she left on my phone.

Two months after her death I made my first New Years resolution ever. It was to be more altruistic and to help others whenever I could. This was meaningful for me since I had been so focused on helping my wife, being there for her and enjoying her company that I was not ever thinking about helping others. I've had several opportunities to assist others in need since that time and it never feels like I'm "giving of myself" since I seem to get more back.

Our house always smelled wonderful, partly since Carolyn usually had a candle burning somewhere in the house. I've never been one to light candles unless there is a power outage. I light them now several times a week to continue keeping the house smelling good, but mostly to remember her and feel close to her. The sense of smell is excellent for triggering those nice thoughts and memories.

In her last year, for my birthday what I wanted was a cordless vacuum since I was starting to take over some of the household duties that she usually took care of. The beauty of this is that I never have to deal with cords and plugs, but the main thing is that the vacuum only lasts for six minutes on a charge and I always have that much time. As a result I vacuum almost every day, which is good since I have 4 pets. Carolyn loved animals, and it was totally her doing that I now have three cats (Red, Beemer & Manny) and our dog Dillon. These animals have been as much a comfort to me as they were for Carolyn when she was feeling sick or down. I see a little of her in each one of the animals and I love them like she did and probably spoil them just as much.

Four months after her death, I was snowboarding at Loveland, a local ski area and feeling a bit guilty actually, since I was in what I call "selfish Chris" mode. This means that I'm just doing whatever I want to do with no accountability to anyone, just myself. Like the song goes, "I'm free to do what I want any old time". I was riding up chair 4 by myself thinking about how much fun snowboarding is. In fact I was giggling when carving turns down the slope. It was that fun. I had quit boarding when we started chemo since Carolyn could not ski due to the osteoporosis and I just wanted to be with her all the time. The joy and beauty that I was feeling from snowboarding made me think of the joy I felt just being with Carolyn and was a strange sort of déjà vu. Good thing I was alone, because tears were flowing down and freezing on my face from happiness and sadness both. Man my emotions are still screwed up.

It's funny but I have started whitewater kayaking much more and it is just a total escape for me. I have to be totally focused on the moment and it is every bit as giggly fun as snowboarding, but without the time to think on the lift. It is also a social activity, which is very helpful.

When I rode the motorcycle for the first time, it just did not feel comfortable or normal. I realized that Carolyn is not on the back patting me on the thigh when we would pass something cool, talking into my ear and giving me the occasional squeeze that lets me know that she is with me and having a good time. I do have a cool patch that I designed for our memorial ride, so I'm always carrying that part of her with me on my rides.

I did not plan on it, but I've lost 20 pounds in the six months since she has been gone. Part of it is that I quit eating sugar at that time; another part is that I can now spend more time (Selfish Chris again) thinking more about my health. In fact I just had hernia surgery that I never really though about before since it seemed so trivial compared to cancer.

I don't want to wait until I'm over Carolyn to get on my life and put this chapter behind me. It is not possible to wait until "I'm over Carolyn", since I'll never be over her, I don't want to be over her and I will truly love her till the day I die. Carolyn was the love of my life, but now that I know it is possible to find true love with your best friend and soul mate. I know it is a long shot, but it should be possible again.

It is some measure of comfort to know that you are not alone in the feelings of grief. Hailey (her daughter) and I still talk to each other when we have tough days. In fact some of Carolyn's girlfriends talk to me about the grief they are still feeling. As time passes, these moments of grief get less and less frequent. That is all part of the healing process. I am so at peace with my life and stronger from having had what I consider a great love. I can only wish the same for others. It is like finding a rare jewel that you carry with you everywhere; only to have it fall out of your pocket years later but just the memory of it makes you feel good.

Fear not, for I am with you;

be not dismayed, for I am your God

-Isaiah 41:10

We are here for only a moment, visitors

and strangers in the land as our ancestors

were before us.

-Chronicles 29:15